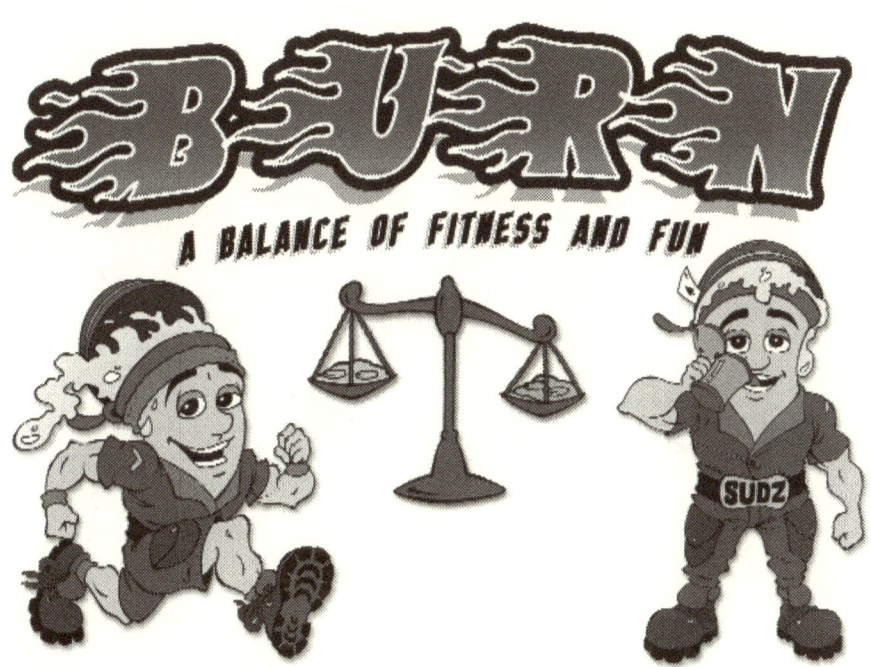

ED MOORE

TRAFFORD

BURN: A Balance of Fitness and Fun
Ed Moore

Note for Librarians: A cataloguing record for this book is available from Library and Archives Canada at www.collectionscanada.ca/amicus/index-e.html
ISBN 1-4251-0308-1

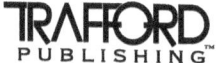

PUBLISHING™
Offices in Canada, USA, Ireland and UK

Book sales for North America and international:
Trafford Publishing, 6E–2333 Government St.,
Victoria, BC V8T 4P4 CANADA
phone 250 383 6864 (toll-free 1 888 232 4444)
fax 250 383 6804; email to orders@trafford.com
Book sales in Europe:
Trafford Publishing (UK) Limited, 9 Park End Street, 2nd Floor
Oxford, UK OX1 1HH UNITED KINGDOM
phone +44 (0)1865 722 113 (local rate 0845 230 9601)
facsimile +44 (0)1865 722 868; info.uk@trafford.com
Order online at:
trafford.com/06-2065

10 9 8 7 6 5 4 3 2 1

Preface

***B**urn: A Balance of Fitness and Fun.*
Sometimes a book title can mislead. Especially this title with its illustration, in which the scale seems to be heavily tipped to the "fun" side.

The truth is that following the program in this book will require lots of training and little fun—until you reach the last two chapters. At that point, all your hard work and effort will begin to pay off. Your level of fitness will allow you to enjoy the day and your surroundings as you glide along your favorite trail. Maybe you will even be able to relish a little competition on the weekend, followed by a couple of cold beers with friends after the race. At that point, the reward will far outweigh the effort.

A word about Private Sudz: he is the mascot for a company that sells drinking products and party paraphernalia (www.beersudz.com), a happy guy who trains hard and enjoys a beer at the end of the day. He is always smiling and upbeat. He keeps his training goals in perspective with the rest of his life.

Let Private Sudz be your inspiration. Sudz is the balance you want to achieve, a serous exercise schedule, followed by equal amounts of relaxation and recovery. Approach your training seriously but don't forget to have fun. Stay focused; don't over-train. The results will be noticeable and gratifying.

As Private Sudz would say: "Cheers!"

Ed Moore
January 2007

About the Author

Ed Moore has been running, exercising, and trying to eat properly for more than forty years. As a result of this consistent effort, his physique is similar to what it was when he was twenty—maybe even a bit better. A retired airline pilot, Ed has figured out where to run—and tested running routes—all over the world. He is the author of two books about running—*The Great American Runner's Guide, Eastern and Western editions.* These books were distributed by *Runner's World* magazine for several years. *The Los Angeles Times* published Ed's running maps during the 1984 Summer Olympics.

Acknowledgments

Thanks to all who helped in the development, design, and production of *Burn!*

Maile and Cassie Moore, my daughters, both university graduates in health and nutrition, helped with the nutrition section.

Lesley Goffinet, massage therapist, contributed to the stretching and injury sections.

Leif Olson and Adam Allison (Hoss Designs) illustrated the book.

Jim Hayes (Cenozoic Design) digitized and revised the city maps.

Heather Bennett (Hither & Yon Publishing Services) managed editorial production.

Introduction

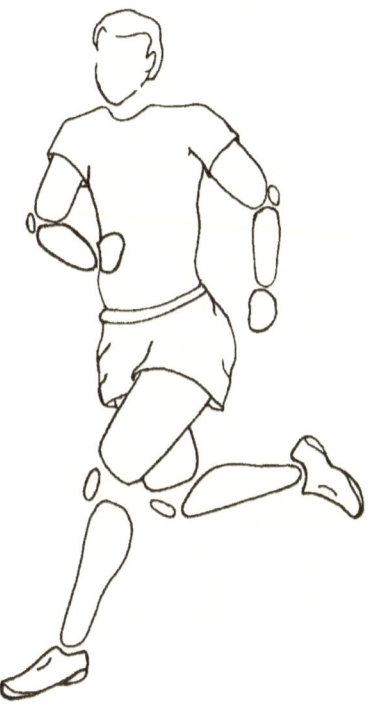

Burn calories! Despite claims to the contrary, there is only one way to lose weight, tone your body, and stay fit. Burn more calories than you consume. Period.

In the scientific world, a calorie is the amount of energy required to heat one milliliter of water one degree centigrade. We use it to measure the work done by muscles in certain activities. For example, you expend approximately 100 calories to walk a mile (270–550 calories per hour).

Most people need 2500 calories to run their bodies for one day—any calories consumed in excess of that number are stored as fat.

I advocate eating, but I also recommend a nutritious diet. If you keep a careful and honest record, you may be surprised at all the empty calories you are eating—calories that contribute little to your nutritional needs and must either be burned through exercise or stored as fat.

There is no easy solution or quick diet fix to get you in shape. Diet fads and pills will not work. You know the truth. You must accept it and commit yourself to change. You will have to change your lifestyle. If you want to get the weight off and your body in shape, exercise must become a part of your daily routine.

But do not despair. If you follow the simple plan outlined in this book, you will soon look forward to getting out there, sweating, and burning off calories. You will meet other people who are dedicated to a lifestyle that includes exercise. You will be able to share these new experiences and discover an inner strength you didn't know you possessed. And you will discover how much fun it is to be healthy.

The positive effects of fitness are not reserved for the professional athlete or the Olympian. Anyone who takes the time and puts forth the effort can use exercise to achieve weight control and health.

Don't let yourself think of exercise as something impossibly difficult. This will prevent you from taking the time to explore its benefits. You are not going to begin with wind sprints and the 100-yard low hurdles. You will gradually work up to your goals and you can jump into my program at any point that feels comfortable. The main objective is to get you out there "burning" and enjoying it.

I do not promise it will be easy. There are no shortcuts to being and staying in good health and reasonable shape. I'm not about to tell you that on five minutes a day you will achieve a washboard stomach or great buns. That does not happen.

After reading this book and following my suggestions, you may love me or hate me; it's really up to you. If you hate me right away you are probably not putting your heart into the program. If you hate me later you're probably searching for a scapegoat to get yourself out of working hard. In either case, try cutting back; then slowly work your way toward more intensity.

You don't need to hate me, but do you need to love yourself—your future body, your new sense of worth and your overall well-being. If this is not the way you feel, step back and evaluate where you are and where you are going. Maybe you have set up too difficult a schedule too early in your training. Make some adjustments and see if you don't feel better.

Another thing that could be discouraging is the fact that you may be expecting results too soon. Take your time. The results will come as long as you put forth the effort. Remember this is not an overnight fix; it's a long-term commitment.

You may experience an initial weight loss right at the beginning if you follow my advice and drink lots of water. This is part of a normal balancing process—your body adjusting the amount of water it has stored. Most people fail to drink the water they need every day. Once you start drinking enough, your body will let some stored water go. You will notice this as a slight change in your weight. Keep drinking the water and this initial weight loss will stay with you. Then you can start working on weight loss by eliminating stored fat.

Take a good look at yourself and honestly decide what you want to achieve. Do you want to lose weight? Maintain weight? Get stronger? Have more stamina? Once you decide on your specific and general goals, you can become more focused and choose the program that will help you reach them.

Let's take an example: Lose weight. This seems to be the number one choice for most people. First, ask yourself why. Why do I want to lose weight? Do I want to lose weight or does somebody else want me to lose weight? Once you decide who's in charge, you can move on to determining how much to lose.

You have to be realistic. A little at a time is the only way to stay healthy and keep it off in the future. The main objective is to set a goal and make it reasonable. Don't set your goals too high. You will become discouraged and lose interest in the entire program. Success at reaching several smaller goals is a lot more rewarding than struggling to reach one major goal, a goal that is difficult or impossible to achieve. Keep it simple. You will find yourself much more content with your new lifestyle of training and exercise.

Along with your weight loss, you will achieve other, more subtle goals. As you lose weight and become fit, your overall conditioning and stamina will improve. Running five miles in one blast will become simple and relaxing. Your speed will naturally increase to a plateau of comfort. Pushing the pace past that plateau, for race training, will take a bit more dedication. The old saying is "If you can't carry on a conversation while you are running, you are going too fast." (Unless, of course, you are training for speed on the track or "fartleks" on the road.)

In order to take the next step—or stride—your diet must also change for the better. Much of this will be because you have forced yourself to eat more balanced meals. As you train more, your body will tell you that it is craving particular foods. In a very real way, it knows what it needs to stay healthy. You need to listen. A good balance of fats, proteins, and carbohydrates will give you energy you never believed you could possess. The vitamins included in that food will satisfy all your daily requirements for a well balanced diet.

Your overall outlook on life should also become more positive and directed. You will feel good about yourself and what you are accomplishing. Little things that used to burden you won't seem to carry the same urgency. You will definitely be better able to cope with everyday ups and downs on a more even keel. Tasks that require exertion, aside from your training, will be easier to achieve. Walking up stairs, playing ball with your kids, going for a swim or bike ride—all will be much simpler. Your respiratory and muscular systems will have changed enough that you can perform these activities using a stronger, more efficient machine—your new body.

Once you start to notice changes in your physique and overall appearance, other changes will already have taken place internally—invisible changes. Your entire system can be overhauled. The food you consume by following this program has so many benefits. You will wonder how you missed them for so many years.

Your heart rate and blood pressure should come down as you progress further into the program. The ratio of HDL (good cholesterol) to LDL (bad cholesterol) should improve as you increase your HDL through exercise.

You'll be well along the road to a happy, healthy existence. Each individual will notice unique, subtle changes. This will make you grin and make you want to tell someone so they can join you in this long-term, rewarding series of changes leading to a more productive life.

Enjoy the journey!

Apparel

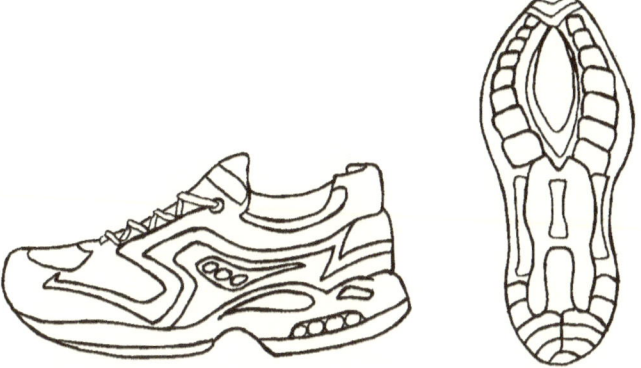

During this first couple of days of shopping I want you to keep a log of what you eat. We will refer back to it. Be honest and record every-thing.

The sport of running doesn't require a tremendous amount of equip-ment. The bare essentials are shoes, shirt, and shorts. With these, you are out the door. Environmental conditions like sun, snow, and wind will dictate what items you'll have to add to this short list. Even some of these items won't break the bank, unless you opt for the designer outfits. Keep in mind that designer clothing is probably better suited for the grocery store or lounging. You won't have to worry about lounging stylishly anymore because you are joining the ranks of active athletes intent on "burning" calories not accumulating them.

Shoes will be your most expensive—and your most important—pur-chase. Don't search for your shoes at the local discount store; you'll definite-ly regret that decision. Make your selection from one of the well-known run-ning stores in your area. Most malls will have Footlocker or Athlete's Foot—or you may find a locally owned store that can provide all the expertise and quality you will require. Take some time with this investment; if you don't it will come back to haunt you in the form of blisters, discomfort, and, in some cases, injuries that will slow your progress and could cost you in med-ical expenses.

Talk to everyone you know who is involved in fitness. Always try to pick a salesperson who is knowledgeable and preferably a runner. The selection of shoes is huge and a high price tag doesn't necessarily mean a great shoe.

You are looking for a comfortable shoe that fits you properly. Let the salesperson know where you are in your training program—beginner, walker, or just recreational. Any information you offer will help the salesperson help you select the correct shoe.

Take you time. Try on both shoes in the pair and walk around the store. Some stores have an area where you can actually jog a little and a few will let you take them for a short run outside. By the time you return for your second pair, you will have a better understanding and feel for the shoe you need.

Running shoes don't last as long as they look like they should. After a few months, the inside of any shoe will be broken down, even if you stayed clear of the mud and the outside appearance is still snazzy. The heel area especially takes a beating and will not be visibly apparent. Old, worn out shoes can ultimately cause quite a few injuries and strained muscles. The average life of a running shoe is about 400–500 miles. This could be stretched a little further if you walk some of your miles. Don't push it. Doctor bills and the frustration of not running will far exceed the cost of new shoes.

Bring your old shoes with you so the salesperson can analyze the wear pattern of your shoe and determine how you are planting your foot when you run. An experienced seller should be able to tell whether you are over or under pronating. Pronating is a word used to describe how your foot rolls when it strikes the ground. Over-pronating your foot exaggerates its natural inward roll and under-pronating (supinating) your foot may cause it to roll to the outside. Knowing whether you are over- or under-pronating will help you select a shoe with the proper heel support to stabilize your foot plant. Be patient and get the shoe that fits your form.

One thing you may encounter when you return for your next pair of shoes—especially if you like your present shoes—is the fact that manufacturers discontinue, change, and upgrade their shoe models often. Once in a while you may be able to buy the same shoe twice in a row, but don't count on it. Some changes will be minor; you can adapt readily. Others will be radical; you may have to switch to a different style or change brands.

Don't get swept away by the high priced models because they aren't necessarily the best shoes, especially for beginners. There are quite a few shoes in the $50–$70 range that should suit you perfectly. Later on in your running program you may want to experiment with a more advanced, full-featured, and therefore pricey shoe—just to see if it really does enhance your running.

I mentioned that weather could influence your selection of appropriate apparel. If you're running outdoors, don't forget the sunscreen—warm or cold, cloudy or clear.

In warm weather, you'll need little more than a cotton t-shirt, shorts, and a visor or hat. Beyond these basics, water—and plenty of it—should be your biggest concern on a hot or humid day.

Cold weather will require a few more items. Lightweight warm-up pants and a jacket will be sufficient in most cases to protect you from the cold and wind. Put on your hat and gloves to keep some of the heat in. Not only are the lightweight warm-up suits easier to run in, they are equally easy to pack when you travel. Most of these items are 100% nylon with 100% polyester lining, which allows them to dry out quickly. This is nice when it comes time to pack for your return trip.

Modern fabrics are designed to move the moisture you create as you run, away from your skin, and at the same time keep your body heat in. Dressing in layers maximizes their effectiveness. The layer closest to your skin, which is usually polypropylene, should be somewhat form fitting. The outer layer should be loose fitting and is often made of nylon or Gore-tex. The inner layer keeps you warm and relatively dry while the outer layer protects you from wind, rain, and other uncomfortable conditions.

Socks, athletic supporter, sports bra, and shorts are all items you will probably want to consider. They are matters of personal preference and comfort; if you are comfortable, you'll perform well. Socks should be lightweight and not cotton. Cotton socks tend to retain moisture so that they bunch up in your shoe and cause blisters and black toenails. Your best choice will be polyester, nylon acrylic, or Lycra.

A runner's watch will be necessary for normal runs and track workouts. Casio makes a reliable watch for about $15.00 that seems to last forever.

Keeping a log is a good idea. This way you can record your daily activities, refer back to them, and chart your progress. Little things provide positive reinforcement. The log is good for checking your results, but you can also use it to plan ahead, so you know when and what you will be doing. Not only is it interesting and fun to go back and read your log, it could also become useful in determining the cause of an injury. You might notice that you added too much mileage in one week or added hills without gradually moving into them. I hope you will only be reviewing it for the pleasant memories.

See page nine for a sample log.

Along with your log, you should also be keeping a planner. Plan your week ahead of time to fit your schedule. Avoiding last-minute adjustments will make your days quite a bit easier.

This is not to say that you can't make small changes once you have started. You don't ever want to feel that you must slavishly carry out a pre-planned workout. If you have planned to run track repeats, but you're feeling particularly sluggish, it's probably not a good idea to continue with that day's conditioning. You have to feel comfortable making changes that fit your mood, while trying to stick to your basic plan. On a sluggish day, switch over to a short run in pleasant surroundings and substitute your track day into another session.

A few other items you'll look forward to buying are new pants, shorts, swimsuits, and other garments as your waistline slowly shrinks. Throw your old clothes away so that, if you return to your sedentary life, you won't have anything to wear. Don't worry. You won't want to go back.

Don't attempt this program in Army boots like Private Sudz!

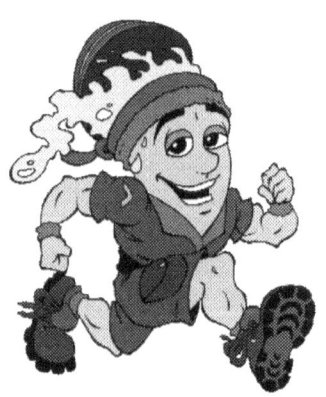

Daily Exercise Log

Use this log to record your daily training.

Date	Location	Distance	Time	Comments
Monday:				
Tuesday:				
Wed.				
Thursday:				
Friday:				
Saturday:				
Sunday:				
		Total:		

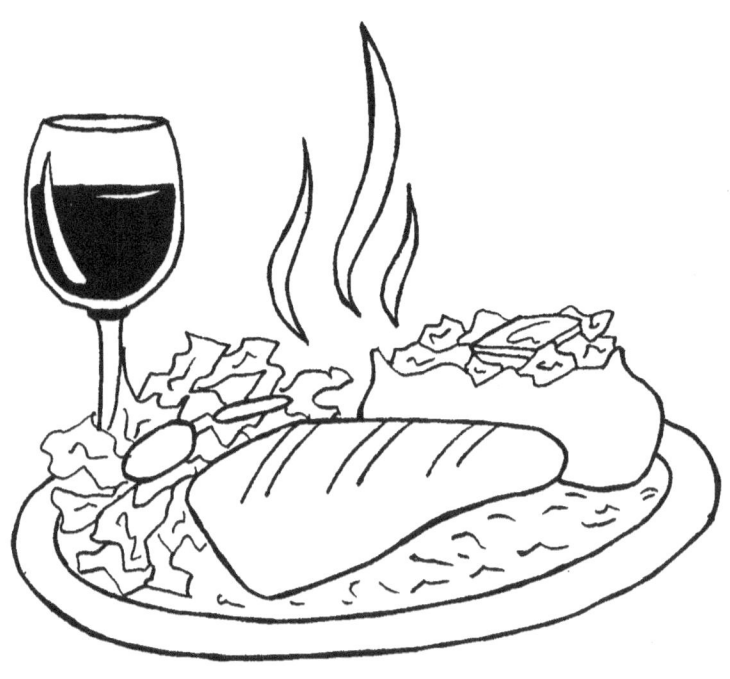

Food & Vitamins

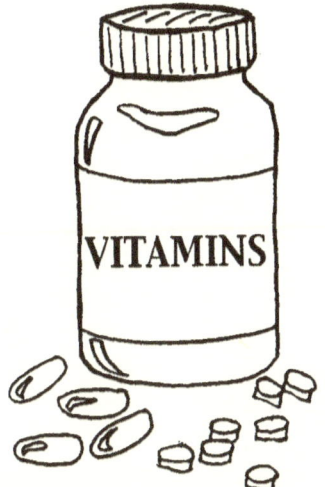

Couch potatoes tend to neglect their eating habits. Nutrition should become as important to you as your workout program. Seek insight into what you eat and how it affects your overall bodily function. "You are what you eat" is basic truth. Changing what and how much you eat will definitely spark other changes.

Once you start a rigorous exercise routine, your diet should begin to change as well. Your body will let you know what it needs—if you listen to it. Schedules are difficult to maintain, but my advice is try to get your exercise done in the morning.

Starting the day with a good breakfast should be one of your first priorities. The way you set up your schedule will dictate when you have your meals. If you are an early riser, you may want to grab a cup of coffee and head for your running trail. You can enjoy a nutritious breakfast when you return. For me, breakfast, is always better after a good run. Others may have a slower start and save their exercise for later in the morning. A good breakfast could begin your day and a good run before lunch will work just fine.

Saving your exercise for the afternoon or early evening generally presents more difficulties. Things happen during the course of any given day that tend to upset your schedule. Pretty soon the exercise you had planned is pushed to the wayside. Another disadvantage of saving your workout for later in the day is that you may be hungry after running and thus over-eat at dinner. This is not a good plan. You don't want to be sleeping on a full stomach.

Before discussing the food and vitamins you should be eating, I'll mention how important drinking water and other liquids will become. The first thing you should know is that you must replenish your body with water—lots of water. Don't wait until you are thirsty; that's too late. As soon as you start drinking water your cells aren't as worried that you are going to dehydrate them and they start releasing stored water. You will notice this drop in weight, which will stabilize as you establish your normal exercise routine. Subsequent weight loss won't be as dramatic, but more consistent.

When you are replenishing after a workout, you might also try some sports drinks, along with water. Sports drinks are absorbed more quickly into your system than solid foods and they can provide the minerals necessary for proper electrolytic balance. A few examples of these drinks are Gatorade, Powerade, All Sport, and Perform. Calorie content varies from 50 in Gatorade to 80 in Powersurge. New drinks called "fitness waters" contain only 10 calories and provide sodium, potassium, B vitamins, and the antioxidant C and E.

You probably don't have to worry too much about salt replenishment because there is so much salt in our American diet. You can sweat 1–2 liters per hour and in that sweat you will lose approximately 1300 milligrams of salt—less than half a teaspoon—and 230 milligrams of potassium.

In moderation, caffeine can also benefit your performance. The scientific explanation is that caffeine helps you burn fat for energy sooner and allows you to save your stored carbohydrates for later. The downside is that caffeine can also raise blood pressure and cause problems during pregnancy. Other effects include aggravating ulcers by increasing acid in the stomach and stimulating bowel activity. This increased bowel activity could work in your favor by cleaning out your system before a run. I wouldn't recommend more than two cups of java daily—mild stimulation without unraveling your nerves.

In the section on apparel, I asked you to write down all the food you ate during the few days you were purchasing your running gear. You know what is good for you and what is bad, but you probably don't know why. I don't want to overwhelm you with scientific data, but I do want to give you information that will enable you to make better choices.

Choosing the right foods and experimenting with different recipes can be fun and rewarding. Getting yourself back in the kitchen and out of the fast food line will make a tremendous difference. Your new diet will make you healthier; it will also give you more energy to continue with your exercise program. You can't run very far on empty calories from the lost trail of junk food junkies.

Speaking of empty calories, let's take a look at the list of food you consumed during your shopping days. The results probably don't surprise you. Now, is that the way you want to continue to eat? I surely hope not.

CALORIC COMPONENTS

As you are now in the business of burning calories, you probably have some idea where these calories originate. All of our food falls into three groups: protein, fat, and carbohydrates. These three groups, added together, comprise the calories consumed on any given day. The trick is to balance these groups in our diets, so that we get the benefits from eating—and enjoy eating at the same time.

Many nutritionists suggest that we try to balance our consumption at 60% carbohydrates, 15% proteins, and 25% fats. If we stick to these proportions and limit our portions at each meal, we will be healthier.

The first advice I offer is incredibly simple: eat slowly and enjoy your meal. If you take the time to savor your foods, you will tend to eat less and not over-stuff your body. The more you eat, the more you have to burn before it goes to fat, so reduce the degree of difficulty: Eat smaller portions of good food and burn some of that stored fat.

CARBOHYDRATES

Let's look at carbohydrates first. There are three types of carbohydrate: simple, complex, and fiber. Simple carbohydrates, often called "carbs" are made of single sugars, glucose being the main one. Glucose is the fuel we run on. Complex carbs are made up of double sugars and have to be broken down by the liver into glucose.

In general, you should try to eat more complex carbs than simple carbs. A few examples of complex carbs include pasta, potato, and rice. A few carbohydrates that have both simple and complex elements are bananas, carrots, and oranges. Purely simple carbs that should be avoided include soft drinks.

Simple carbs tend to boost insulin levels—much more dramatically than do complex carbs. Insulin locks fat in and protects it from being burned for energy.

Complex carbohydrates are stored in the liver and muscles as glycogen. Replenish your system with carbohydrates soon after you exercise to help reload your glycogen stores. The sooner you eat the better. If you fail to replenish glycogen, your workouts will become more and more difficult and you become more vulnerable to muscle strain and injury.

Fiber is another form of carbohydrate that contains no calories. In fact, the body doesn't digest fiber at all. Instead of being absorbed, it passes through the system as bulk. Sources of fiber include fruits, vegetables, nuts, and whole grains.

FATS

Fats fall into three groups: saturated, monounsaturated, and polyunsaturated. Each group contains both healthful and unhealthful properties. Fat carries fat-soluble vitamins (A, D, E, and K) and some dietary fat is essential to maintain the proper function of human cells, particularly nerve cells. Fat is also directly associated with two words we commonly hear when discussing health and diets—cholesterol and calories.

Fats tend to be high in calories. Cutting down on fat consumption automatically reduces calorie intake.

All animal fats contain cholesterol and cholesterol is the chief ingredient in our cells walls. The trick is knowing how much and what kind of cholesterol is floating in our blood. Low-density lipoproteins (LDL) carry cholesterol in the general circulation and high-density lipoproteins (HDL) carry cholesterol on it way out of the system. Therefore HDL is considered the "good cholesterol" and LDL the "bad cholesterol."

Exercise tends to increase the presence of HDL. Red wine is also good for your HDL levels because it contains flavinoids, which are found in the skin of red grapes.

Most dairy and meat products contain saturated fats: butter, cheese, and ice cream are a few examples. A diet high in saturated fats—especially in the absence of exercise—has been shown to elevate LDL and promote heart disease.

Monounsaturated fats seem to be healthier. Monounsaturates can be found in one of my favorite foods, avocado, as well as in olive and canola oils.

Trans fats, or "transfatty acids," are formed in the process of "hydrogenating" oil, typically vegetable oil. Fats have long carbon chains. Unsaturated fats—both monounsaturates and polyunsaturates—break down rather easily, so hydrogen is added to make them more stable, giving fat-based food a longer shelf life. This process produces trans fats. Trans fats are found in anything that contains hydrogenated vegetable oil, partially hydrogenated vegetable oil, or vegetable shortening. The FDA now requires trans fat amounts to be listed in the nutrition information on food labels.

Margarine, potato chips, and cookies are good examples of food choices containing polyunsaturated fat. These foods are, in most cases, not good for you and hard to digest. They should be avoided. Trans fats have been shown to increase LDL (bad cholesterol) and heart disease and may increase your chances of developing some cancers.

Omega-3 fats have great health benefits. These fats reduce the chances of blood clots and therefore stroke. The best sources of omega -3 are anchovies, herring, sardines, salmon, whitefish, tuna, mackerel, and striped bass.

Your genes may ultimately determine your blood cholesterol levels, but your diet is also a big contributor. By simply decreasing or eliminating your consumption of fried foods, you can improve your ratio of LDL to HDL. Most fried foods contain partially hydrogenated fat, which increases the amount of LDL in your system. Cut back on the crackers and chips.

PROTEINS

Proteins are broken down into amino acids, which are necessary in building and repairing body tissue, defending against disease, and promoting growth. Overeating proteins won't be of much benefit because your body can't store proteins without converting them to fat. Right after exercise, you will benefit from eating some proteins, along with the carbohydrates, to get the muscle re-building process started.

Keep in mind a few numbers while you study the following food lists and their breakdown into carbohydrates, fats, proteins, and total calories. One gram of either carbohydrate or protein contributes 4 calories while fat contributes more than twice as many—9 calories.

1 gram carbohydrate = 4 calories

1 gram protein = 4 calories

1 gram fat = 9 calories

Don't be surprised if you see numbers that differ from mine. I tried to figure out which values were "correct," but apparently everybody has a different method of determining the final numbers. Nevertheless, most of the conclusions seem to be consistent across multiple sources, so use these tables as a starting point for making your food choices. If you really want to get more involved, which may not be necessary, you can check other books and studies.

NOTE: Good for snacks and energy. You can eat comfortably in this category.

FRUITS	CARBOHYDRATE	FAT	PROTEIN	CALORIES
Apple, 1 med.	20			80
Apricots, 3 med.	11			44
Avocado, 1 med. Haas	12	30	4	334
Banana, 1 med.	26			104
Cantaloupe, 1/2	23			92
Cherries, 1 cup	20		2	88
Grapefruit, 1/2	13		1	56
Grapes, 1-1/2 cup	24	1	1	90
Honeydew, 1 wedge	15		1	64
Kiwi, 1 med.	11		1	48
Orange, 1 med.	17			68
Papaya, 1/2	12	1		52
Peach, 1 med.	9	1		40
Pear, 1 med.	25			100
Pineapple, 2 slices	16	1		68
Raisins, 1/4 cup	31	1		128
Raspberries, 1/2 cup	7	1		32
Strawberries, 1/2 cup	5			20
Watermelon, 1 slice	21	1	3	103

NOTE: These calories are not as good as the fruits, but won't hurt if you continue to "burn" your calories.

BREADS & CEREALS	CARBOHYDRATES	FAT	PROTEINS	CALORIES
White, 1 slice	12	1	2	65
Wheat, 1 slice	14	1	3	77
Cinnamon Raisin	12	1	2	56
Sourdough, 1 slice	15	1	2	77
Rye, 1 slice	14	1	3	77
Bagel, 1 medium	45	1	7	217
Corn bread	20	3	3	119
Croissant	14	5	3	113
Dinner roll	14	2	2	82
English muffin	26	1	4	129
Banana nut muffin	29	7	3	191
French toast, 1 slice	16	5	5	145
Pancakes, 3	40	4	6	220
Oat meal, 1oz/1cup	23	3	5	139
Cornflakes	25		2	108
Raisin Bran, 1 cup	46	1	4	209

NOTE: Vegetables are always good and have the added advantage of more proteins.

VEGETABLES	CARBOHYDRATES	FATS	PROTEINS	CALORIES
Artichoke, 1 medium.	13		4	68
Asparagus, 4 spears	2		1	12
Beans, baked	28	1	7	149
Beans, green, 1/2 cup	5		1	24
Beans, re-fried	18	2	6	114
Broccoli, 1 stalk	9		5	56
Carrot, 1 med.ium	7		1	32
Cauliflower, 1/2 cup	2		1	12
Celery, 1 stalk	1			4
Coleslaw, 1/2 cup	7	1	1	41
Corn, 1/2 cup	19	1	2	93
Corn, cob	28	1	4	137
Cucumber, 1/2 cup	1			7
Lettuce, 4 leaves	1			4
Onions, 1 slice	1			4
Peas, 1/2 cup	10		4	56
Pepper (green or red), 1/2 cup	5		1	24
Potato, Baked	51		5	224
French Fries, 3oz	23	5	2	145
Mashed, 1/2 cup w/butter	18	1	2	89

VEGETABLES	CARBOHYDRATES	FATS	PROTEINS	CALORIES
Hash browns, 3 oz	17		2	76
Scalloped potatos, 1/2 cup	13	4	2	96
Rice, white, 1/2 cup	22		2	96
Rice, brown, 1/2 cup	22		2	100
Spinach, 1/2 cup	3		3	24
Squash, yellow summer. 1/2 cup	4		1	20
Tomato,1 med.	8			36
Zucchini, 1 cup	3		1	16

NOTE: This is where you will get your fat percentage along with proteins. You have to include some fat and lean meats, along with avocado and monounsaturated oils, are the best choices.

MEAT, CHICKEN, FISH	CARBOHYDRATES	FATS	PROTEINS	CALORIES
Ground round beef, 4 oz, 80% lean		22	20	278
Flank steak, 4 oz.		14	30	246
T-bone, 4 oz		25	23	576
Sirloin steak, 4 oz		13	52	317
Bacon, 2 strips		7	5	83
Frankfurter	3	13	5	149
Ham slice	1	1	8	45

Meat, Chicken, Fish	Carbohydrates	Fats	Proteins	Calories
Sausage, 3 oz	2	19	7	207
Veal cutlet		36	11	368
Veal shank		7	36	207
Leg of lamb		19	29	287
Lamb chop		26	28	346
Chicken breast, 1/2		7	29	179
Drumstick w/skin		6	14	110
Turkey breast, no skin		3	34	163
Turkey slice		1	11	48
Sea bass, 4 oz		3	27	135
Catfish		3	21	111
Cod		1	26	113
Halibut		3	30	147
Mahi-mahi		1	27	117
Perch		1	28	121
Salmon		14	25	226
Swordfish		6	29	170
Trout		9	30	201
Tuna		7	34	199
Tuna-canned in water, 2 oz.		1	15	69

Meat, Chicken, Fish	Carbohydrates	Fats	Proteins	Calories
Clams, canned	2		9	44
Crab, steamed		2	22	106
Lobster, steamed	1	1	23	105
Mussels, canned	4	5	11	105
Oysters, raw	3	2	6	54
Scallops, baked	4	5	25	161
Scallops, fried	20	6	9	170
Shrimp, steamed /cooked (4) large			5	20

NOTE: Dairy products are, in many cases, a balance carbs, fats, and proteins. Don't shy away from them; they are good for you. Calcium is plentiful in most dairy items.

Dairy	Carbohydrates	Fats	Proteins	Calories
Fried egg		7	6	87
Egg white			4	16
Boiled egg		5	6	69
Scrambled egg w/milk	1	7	7	95
American cheese, 1 slice	2	5	4	78
Swiss cheese, 1 slice	1	6	4	74
Cheddar cheese, 1 slice		9	7	114
Cottage cheese (2%), 1/2 cup	4	2	15	94

DAIRY	CARBOHYDRATES	FATS	PROTEINS	CALORIES
Butter, 1 tsp		11		99
Margarine		11		99
Cream (half & half), 1 tsp	1	2	1	20
Whole milk	11	8	8	148
2% milk	13	5	8	125
Nonfat milk	12		8	80
Sour cream (lite), 2 tsp	2	2.5	2	39
Lowfat yogurt	17	4	3	262
Vanilla ice cream, 1 cup	30	14	4	270
Chocolate ice cream, 1 cup	34	14	4	278

NOTE: Snacks are fun at parties and special occasions, but don't overdo the chips. Stick to the nuts for better fats.

NUTS & SNACKS	CARBOHYDRATES	FATS	PROTEINS	CALORIES
Almonds, 1/4 cup (28)	6	14	6	174
Cashews, 1/4 cup	9	13	4	109
Macadamia, 1/4 cup	4	21	2	213
Pecans, 1/4 cup	4	21	3	217
Sunflower seeds	6	14	6	174
Walnuts	4	19	4	203

Nuts & Snacks	Carbohydrates	Fats	Proteins	Calories
Peanuts, dry roasted	6	14	8	182
Trail mix, 1/4 cup	14	7	3	131
Popcorn, 1 cup, no salt or oil	6	1	1	37
Pretzel, (17)	24	1	3	117
Frito, 1 oz (15)	9	6	1	94
Potato, 1oz. (15)	15	10	2	158
Tortilla, 1oz. 6-10	18	6	2	134
Wheat thins (16)	20	6	4	42
Bacon flavored (15)	19	8	3	160
Triscuit, reduced fat (7)	21	3	3	123
Town House, reduced fat (6)	11	2	1	66

NOTE: This table is for viewing only. You will not find much useful food here and it is very difficult to "burn" off any excesses.

Desserts	Carbohydrates	Fats	Proteins	Calories
Chocolate chip cookie	11	5	1	87
Oatmeal cookie	16	4	2	100
Oreo cookie	15	5	1	107
Plain doughnut	25	12		210
Sugared doughnut	27	11		220

DESSERTS	CARBOHYDRATES	FATS	PROTEINS	CALORIES
Glazed doughnut	34	12		250
Chocolate doughnut	29	14		260
Danish pastry	26	12	4	220
Angel food cake	29		3	128
Cheesecake	20	18	4	128
Apple pie, 1 piece	37	11	2	250
Blueberry pie	32	9	2	270
Pumpkin pie	29	8	5	270
Chocolate cake	41	13	2	289
Pound cake	39	9	4	253

MISCELLANEOUS	CARBOHYDRATES	FATS	PROTEINS	CALORIES
Peanut butter, 2 tsp	6	16	8	190
Honey, 1 tsp	17			65
Syrup, 1 tsp	13			52
Jam, 1 tsp	14			55
Catsup, 1 tsp	4			15
Mayonnaise, 1 tsp		11		100
Salsa, 2 tsp	2			8

MISCELLANEOUS	CARBOHYDRATES	FATS	PROTEINS	CALORIES
Miracle Whip (lite), 1 tsp	3	2		30
Miracle Whip	2	4		44

NOTE: Fat-free and you are home free. A nice salad with vegetables and fat-free dressing will curb your appetite in a good way.

SALAD DRESSING	CARBOHYDRATES	FATS	PROTEINS	CALORIES
Blue cheese	2	16		150
Caesar	2	14		140
French	5	11		150
Ranch	3	18		180
1000 island	5	12		130
FAT FREE				
Balsamic Vinaigrette	6			24
Blue cheese	9			36
Caesar	8			32
Honey Dijon	10			40
Italian	4			16
Ranch	7			28
Thousand Island	10		1	44
French	11			44

DRINKS, JUICE	CARBOHYDRATES	FATS	PROTEINS	CALORIES
Apple, 8 oz	28			112
Grape, 8 oz	34			136
Orange, 8 oz	26		1	108
Pineapple, 8 oz	30			120
Tomato V-8, 8 oz	11		2	52
Lemonade, 8 oz	24			96

NOTE: Water should be your "soft" drink of preference.

DRINKS, SODA	CARBOHYDRATES	FATS	PROTEINS	CALORIES
Coke, 12 oz	28			112
Root beer, 12 oz	31			124
7-Up, 12 oz	26			84
Ginger Ale, 12 oz	21			84
Pepsi, 12 oz	27			108

NOTE:: A cold beer in the evening or at a sporting event has always been one of my weaknesses. Especially "micro brews."

DRINKS, ALCOHOL	CARBOHYDRATES	FATS	PROTEINS	CALORIES
Beer, 12 oz	13		1	146
Light beer, 12 oz	5		1	99
Vodka etc., 1 oz				82
Red wine, 3 oz	2			74
White wine, 3 oz	1			70

DRINKS, COFFEE	CARBOHYDRATES	FATS	PROTEINS	CALORIES
Latte	17	11	11	210

NOTE: Here are some statistics on common meals and soups.

MEALS & SOUPS	CARBOHYDRATES	FATS	PROTEINS	CALORIES
Chilli con carne, 1 cup	38	13	20	349
Chilli with beans, 1 cup	26	11	17	270
Lasagna	41	10	18	326
Spaghetti	50	6	10	294
Chicken noodle soup	8	2	4	66
Chicken rice soup	13	1	2	69
Tomato soup	20		2	88
Vegetable beef soup	15	1	5	88
New England clam chowder	13	3	4	95
Manhattan clam chowder	12	2	2	74

NOTE:: Turn the page. You'll find a list of some places you used to frequent, along with calorie counts for those foods you don't eat any more. Compare these numbers to the ones above and you'll see why fast food visits no longer fit into your new schedule! Save the calories for those microbreweries you'll encounter on your journeys.

Fast Food	Carbohydrates	Fats	Proteins	Calories
Burger King Whopper	53	40	29	680
Wendy's Classic	37	19	25	410
McDonald's Big Mac	47	34	24	590
Domino's pizza, thin crust	31	12	12	273
Domino's pizza, thick crust	68	27	23	598
Taco Bell taco	18	12	9	216

VITAMINS

Eating good food should give you all the vitamins and antioxidants you require, but it doesn't hurt to add a few supplements to fill in what may be missing or under-represented in your diet. One term needs explanation: antioxidant.

Like rust on a car, oxidation can cause damage to cells. antioxidant exist as vitamins, minerals, and other compounds in foods. They may help boost immune response and decrease the risk of infection and cancer, though scientists are not in agreement about their effectiveness.

Antioxidants include carotenoids, which gives fruits and vegetables their rich colors. Vitamin C and E are good antioxidants, as well as, magnesium, copper, and zinc.

I will mention a few of the more important vitamins you should try to consume daily—either through your diet or with supplements. Many vitamins interact with each other. You would be wise to discuss your vitamin intake with your doctor or pharmacist to be sure you're getting the proper doses.

FAT-SOLUBLE VITAMINS

The first group of vitamins is fat soluble. These vitamins can be stored in the liver and in fat tissue. If you take too much of these vitamins, you could build up to a toxic level. Don't over do it. Stick with the recommended daily allowances (RDA) dosages. Vitamin A can be toxic in large amounts.

VITAMIN A

This is stored in the liver. It is also an antioxidant and is thought to help protect against infection. It's good for vision and counteracts night blindness. This vitamin maintains the epithelial cells, which make up your skin and the membranes lining your mouth and the length of your intestines, respiratory, and reproductive passages.

Sources of vitamin A

Liver	Sweet potatoes
Fish oils	Carrots
Egg yolks	Squash
Milk	Apricots
Leafy green vegetables	Cantaloupes

VITAMIN E (TOCOPHEROL)

This vitamin is another important antioxidant that protects cell membranes from destruction by free radicals, which helps to keep you younger looking and alleviates fatigue. Vitamin E aids in the formation of red blood cells and in healing. Vitamin E should be taken along with vitamin A to help in the absorption of vitamin A.

Sources of vitamin E

Wheat germ	Soybeans
Liver or Eggs	Brussels sprouts
Whole grain	Spinach
Vegetable oils	Green leafy vegetables

Nuts and seeds (almonds, peanuts, cashews, and sunflower seeds)

VITAMIN D

This vitamin is good for healthy bones and teeth and also crucial for the absorption of dietary calcium. Along with A and C, it will help in preventing colds.

Vitamin D is manufactured by the body when the body is exposed to sunlight for approximately 15 minutes.

Food sources of vitamin D

Milk	Liver
Cheese	Sardines
Egg yolk	Tuna
Cod liver oil	Salmon

VITAMIN K

This vitamin encourages normal blood clotting.

Sources of vitamin K

Turnip greens	Whole grains	Cod liver oil
Leafy vegetables	Green tea	
Egg yolk	Soybean oil	

WATER-SOLUBLE VITAMINS

You can't overdose on a water-soluble vitamin. If you take too much of one of these vitamins, the excess is extracted by the kidneys and excreted in the urine.

The major vitamin in this category is vitamin B. Vitamin B is made of several different groups, which is why it is easier to take a multi-vitamin B.

THIAMIN (VITAMIN B1)

Thiamine is needed for carbohydrates to release energy. It aids in digestion of carbohydrates, fats, and proteins, plus normal functioning of the heart and nervous system.

Sources of vitamin B1

Pork	Whole grains
Liver	Milk
Legumes	Meat
Fish	Nuts
Poultry	Potatoes
Eggs	

RIBOFLAVIN (VITAMIN B2)

Riboflavin facilitates metabolism and energy release from carbohydrates, fats, and proteins, healthy skin, and linings of the digestive system and the lungs. It also benefits vision and prevent eye fatigue.

Sources of vitamin B2

Liver	Broccoli
Milk	Avocados
Cheese	Brussels sprouts
Meats	Eggs
Seafood	Green leafy vegetables
Asparagus	

NIACIN (VITAMIN B3)

Niacin is needed for normal cell metabolism and energy release from carbohydrates. It adds to synthesis of hormones and DNA. It acts like vitamin Bl and B2 in normal cell metabolism to release energy from carbohydrates, fats, and proteins. It also improves circulation of blood and reduces cholesterol and triglycerol levels.

Sources of vitamin B3

Organ meat	Poultry
Fish	Dates
Figs	Nuts
Green vegetables	Legumes
Whole-wheat cereals	Avocado

PANTOTHENIC ACID (VITAMIN B5)

B5 supports energy release from carbohydrates, fats, and proteins and aids synthesis of adrenal hormones and chemicals involved in the nervous system.

Sources of vitamin B5

Organ meats	Milk products
Egg yolks	Mushrooms
Nuts	Green vegetables
Whole grains	Poultry

PYRIDOXINE (VITAMIN B6)

B6 supports protein metabolism and helps in metabolizing carbohydrates and fats. It increases the production of serotonin, which elevates mood and increases a calm, positive feeling. It also helps damaged nerve cells regenerate.

Sources of vitamin B6

Blackstrap molasses	Meat (steak)
Organ meats	Poultry
Wheat germ	Brewers yeast
Whole grains	Fish
Soybeans	Bananas
Avocado	Green leafy vegetables
Peanuts	Melon

FOLIC ACID (VITAMIN B9)

B9 helps in making red blood cells and genetic material (DNA and RNA).

Sources of vitamin B9 (folic acid)

Green leafy vegetables	Organ meats
Legumes	Orange juice
Beets	Avocados
Broccoli	Carrots

VITAMIN B12

Along with folic acid, B12 helps to form red blood cells. It supports a healthy nervous system. Too much vitamin C could reduce the ability to absorb B12 from your food.

Sources of vitamin B12

Meat	Liver
Poultry	Fish
Shellfish	Eggs
Cheese	Milk

VITAMIN C (ASCORBIC ACID)

Vitamin C is an antioxidant. It is needed for healthy gums and healing of wounds. It helps produce collagen and holds cells together. It increases calcium and iron absorption. Too much vitamin C (1000 mg or more) could hinder the absorption of vitamin B12. It helps to prevent the common cold.

Sources of vitamin C

Red peppers	Broccoli
Citrus fruits	Strawberries
Melons	Kiwi
Mangos	Tomatoes
Potatoes	Raw cabbage
Spinach	Turnips
Cauliflower	

BIOTIN

Biotin is used for energy metabolism and synthesis of fats, proteins, and carbohydrates. It lowers blood sugar. It also slows the graying of hair and inhibits baldness.

Sources of Biotin

Organ meat (liver)	Oatmeal
Egg yolk	Milk
Soybeans	Peanuts
Peanut butter	Whole grains
Fruits	Vegetables

MINERALS

Along with vitamins, you should also be ingesting minerals, including calcium, iron, chromium, fluoride, magnesium, manganese, potassium, selenium (antioxidant), and zinc.

CALCIUM

This mineral is very prevalent in the human body and is necessary in maintaining skeletal integrity. As they age, women should be more concerned with proper amounts of calcium in their diets. Loss of bone mass is referred to as osteoporosis. Calcium helps to heal wounds and prevent infection—along with fighting fatigue. It also aids in the contraction of smooth muscles.

Sources of Calcium

Dairy products	Spinach
Broccoli	Cauliflower
Turnip greens	Cabbage
Asparagus	Beans
Nuts	Figs

IRON

This mineral is needed to produce hemoglobin in your blood system. White blood cells also require iron to develop properly. Anemia could result from inadequate iron in the diet.

Sources of Iron

Beef	Liver
Veal	Chicken
Pork	Clams
Eggs	Spinach
Asparagus	Prunes
Raisins	

CHROMIUM

This mineral regulates blood sugar and works with insulin to drive sugar from your blood for use and storage.

Sources of Chromium

Brewer's yeast	Wheat germ
Liver	Meat
Cheese	Legumes
Beans	Peas
Black pepper	

FLUORIDE

The main function of fluoride lies in preventing tooth decay. It will strengthen teeth and bones. Some cities add fluoride to local water supplies.

Sources of Fluoride

Herring	Sardines
Tea	Salmon

MAGNESIUM

This is used in the metabolism of glucose, oxidation of fatty acids, and activation of amino acids. It helps in preventing depression. The balance of calcium to magnesium should be 2 to 1 to allow for the proper absorption. Magnesium is required for relaxation of muscle after contraction.

Sources of Magnesium

Nuts	Legumes
Spinach	Soybeans
Peas	Molasses
Cornmeal	Shrimp
Clams	Oysters
Crab	

MANGANESE

This is used to metabolize fats, and to build bones and connective tissue. It plays a major part in cellular division.

Sources of Manganese

Whole grains	Cereals
Fruits	Green vegetables
Tea	Ginger
Cloves	

POTASSIUM

Potassium helps control nerve impulses and contraction of muscles. Another function is maintaining blood pressure in the normal range.

Sources of Potassium

Dried apricots	Cantaloupe
Lima beans	Potato
Avocado	Bananas
Broccoli	Liver
Milk	Peanut butter
Citrus fruits	

SELENIUM

This mineral works with vitamin E to form an antioxidant called glutathione.

Sources of Selenium

Seafood	Liver
Kidney	

SODIUM

This mineral regulates the balance of water in your body fluids and cells.

Sources of Sodium

Table salt	Soy sauce

ZINC

Zinc promotes the proper growth of hair, skin, and nails. It also helps the immune system to fight colds and other diseases and to heal wounds.

Sources of Zinc

Beef	Liver
Chicken	Oysters
Herring	Clams
Wheat germ	Carrots
Peas	Bran
Oatmeal	Nuts

MENU PLANNING

Skipping meals is not the answer, but eating nutritious meals should be part of your new schedule. Creating a healthier menu should be easier if you refer to the tables I have included below. Concentrate on putting together meals that contain a balance of carbohydrates, fats, and proteins. The majority of vitamins and minerals will be there if you are eating proper food. Remember the proportions of calories in a balanced diet: carbohydrates 60%, proteins 15%, and fats 25%.

Changing your diet will automatically increase the amount of helpful vitamins you consume. You may want to add a few supplements, like the antioxidant E, C, and B. Otherwise, take a look at the list I have laid out, with the benefits each will provide. You can also look at the different food groups and choose the food that contains these vitamins and minerals. You don't have to become a graduate in scientific nutrition to eat properly. For the most part, you know what is good for you and what is putting on the weight. Make the adjustments slowly. As your program progresses, you may want to research a little and refine your eating habits. Right now you have to concentrate on "burning off" whatever you put in your stomach above and beyond the 2500 calories per day average.

With all this new knowledge you can begin to create new choices for your dining pleasure that will not only satisfy your taste buds but replenish the muscles that have been depleted through your new lifestyle of strenuous exercise.

Remember, smaller portions are the best way to eat. No more huge meals; more small ones. A balanced diet, along with plenty of water, will make everything seem easier—not just your exercise program, your everyday life as well. Your mood will improve, as will your general attitude. You will feel good—perhaps for the first time.

The following seven days of meals should be used as examples for your new diet. You may want to reduce total calories a little, until you get further into the "burning" portion of your training.

MONDAY

Food Item	Carbohydrates	Fat	Protein	Calories
BREAKFAST				
Grapefruit (1/2)	13			52
Pancakes (3)	40	4	6	220
Syrup, 2 tsp.	26			104
Tomato juice (V-8)	11		2	52
Coffee				
SNACK				
Peach	9			36
LUNCH				
BLT sandwich	41	17	15	377
Tomato soup	20		2	88
SNACK				
Apple	20			80
DINNER				
Trout		9	30	201
Rice, 1/2 cup	22		2	96
Spinach	1		1	8
Water	ADD	TO	ANY	MEAL!
TOTALS	203 g	30 g	58 g	
	x 4 g/cal	x 9 g/cal	x 4 g/cal	**TOTAL**
	= 812 cal	= 270 cal	= 232 cal	**1314** CAL
% daily intake	62%	21%	17%	
With Beer, 12 oz	13	13 alcohol*	1	148
*There is no fat in beer, but each gram of alcohol averages 7.1 calories. The average beer has 13 grams of alcohol—an extra 92.3 calories.				**TOTAL**
				1462 CAL

TUESDAY

Food Item	Carbohydrates	Fat	Protein	Calories
BREAKFAST				
Papayat (1/2)	12		2	52
Toast	14	1	3	77
Grape juice	34			136
Coffee				
SNACK				
Banana	26			104
LUNCH				
Chili, 1 cup	28	10	22	290
Corn muffin	27	5	2	161
Water	ADD	TO	ANY	MEAL!
SNACK				
Orange	17			68
DINNER				
Salmon, 4 oz		14	25	226
Mashed potato	14	4	2	100
Asparagus	2		1	12
Pear	25			100
TOTALS	199 g	34 g	56 g	
	x 4 g/cal	x 9 g/cal	x 4 g/cal	**TOTAL**
	= 796 cal	= 306 cal	= 224 cal	**1326** CAL
% daily intake	60%	25%	17%	
With Beer, 12 oz	13	13 alcohol*	1	148
*There is no fat in beer, but each gram of alcohol averages 7.1 calories. The average beer has 13 grams of alcohol—an extra 92.3 calories.			**TOTAL**	**1474** CAL

WEDNESDAY

Food Item	Carbohydrates	Fat	Protein	Calories
BREAKFAST				
Strawberries or Raspberries	12		1	52
French toast	20	5	5	145
Syrup, 1 tsp	13			52
Pineapple juice	30			120
SNACK				
Orange	17			68
LUNCH				
Egg white omelette with veggies			12	48
Tomato slices	8			36
Water	ADD	TO	ANY	MEAL!
SNACK				
Carrots	7		1	32
DINNER				
Chick quesadilla	33	26	25	466
Spanish rice, 1/4 c	34	1	3	153
Salad with dressing (non-fat French)	15			60
TOTALS	189 g	32 g	47 g	
	x 4 g/cal	x 9 g/cal	x 4 g/cal	**TOTAL**
	= 756 cal	= 288 cal	= 188 cal	**1232** CAL
% daily intake	60%	25%	17%	
With Beer, 12 oz	13	13 alcohol*	1	148
*There is no fat in beer, but each gram of alcohol averages 7.1 calories. The average beer has 13 grams of alcohol—an extra 92.3 calories.				**TOTAL** **1380** CAL

THURSDAY

FOOD ITEM	CARBOHYDRATES	FAT	PROTEIN	CALORIES
BREAKFAST				
Kiwi	11			44
Wheat toast	14	1	3	77
Orange juice	26			104
SNACK				
Banana	26			104
LUNCH				
Tuna salad	6	5	15	129
Tomato soup with water	18	2	1	74
Frito chips	9	6	1	94
Water	ADD	TO	ANY	MEAL!
SNACK				
Apple	20			80
Cheee slices	2	5	4	69
DINNER				
Flank steak		14	30	246
Rice	41		4	180
Summer squash	8		2	40
TOTALS	181 g	33 g	60 g	
	x 4 g/cal	x 9 g/cal	x 4 g/cal	**TOTAL**
	= 724 cal	= 297 cal	= 240 cal	**1261** CAL
% daily intake	57%	24%	19%	
With Beer, 12 oz	13	13 alcohol*	1	148
*There is no fat in beer, but each gram of alcohol averages 7.1 calories. The average beer has 13 grams of alcohol—an extra 92.3 calories.			**TOTAL**	
			1409 CAL	

FRIDAY

Food Item	Carbohydrates	Fat	Protein	Calories
BREAKFAST				
Honeydew, 1 wedge	15		1	64
Toast	14	1	3	77
Apple juice, 8 oz	28			112
SNACK				
Pear	25			100
LUNCH				
Egg salad sandw.: Bread (2) Eggs (2) Miracle Whip Tomato slice Avacado (1/2)	36 2 4 6	2 10 4 25	8 12 2	194 138 44 16 167
Cottage cheese (2%). 1/2 cup	4	2	15	94
Chicken noodle soup	8	2	4	66
SNACK				
Apple	20			80
DINNER				
Spaghetti	50	6	10	294
Artichoke	13		4	68
Salad with Italian dressing	8			32
TOTALS	221 g	42 g	55 g	
	x 4 g/cal	x 9 g/cal	x 4 g/cal	**TOTAL**
	= 884 cal	= 378 cal	= 220 cal	**1482** CAL
% daily intake	60%	25%	15%	
With Beer, 12 oz	13	13 alcohol*	1	148
*There is no fat in beer, but each gram of alcohol averages 7.1 calories. The average beer has 13 grams of alcohol—an extra 92.3 calories.				**TOTAL** **1630** CAL

SATURDAY

Food Item	Carbohydrates	Fat	Protein	Calories
BREAKFAST				
Grapefruit	13			52
Pancakes (3)	40	4	6	220
Syrup	26			104
SNACK				
Raisins	31			128
LUNCH				
Turkey sandwich	39	6	17	278
Beef vegetable soup	5	3	6	71
Water	Add	to	any	meal!
SNACK				
Carrots	7		1	32
DINNER				
Hamburger patty		22	20	278
Corn on the cob	28	1	4	137
Broccololi, 1 stalk	9		5	56
TOTALS	198 g	36 g	60 g	
	x 4 g/cal	x 9 g/cal	x 4 g/cal	**TOTAL**
	= 792 cal	= 324 cal	= 240 cal	**1356** CAL
% daily intake	59%	24%	17%	
With Beer, 12 oz	13	13 alcohol*	1	148
*There is no fat in beer, but each gram of alcohol averages 7.1 calories. The average beer has 13 grams of alcohol—an extra 92.3 calories.				**TOTAL** **1504** CAL

Food & Vitamins

SUNDAY				
FOOD ITEM	CARBOHYDRATES	FAT	PROTEIN	CALORIES
BREAKFAST				
Cantaloupe, 1/2	23			92
Scrambled egg whites (2)			8	32
Toast	12	1	2	65
Orange juice	26			104
SNACK				
Orange	17			68
LUNCH				
Chicken salad		4	15	96
1000 Island Dressing	11			44
Tomato soup with water	20	2		88
SNACK				
Pear	25			100
DINNER				
Lasagne	41	10	18	326
Pineapple slices (2)	16			68
Salad	2			8
Avocado, 1/2	7	15	2	171
TOTALS	203 g	30 g	49 g	
	x 4 g/cal	x 9 g/cal	x 4 g/cal	**TOTAL**
	= 812 cal	= 270 cal	= 196 cal	**1278** CAL
% daily intake	59%	24%	17%	
With Beer, 12 oz	13	13 alcohol*	1	148
*There is no fat in beer, but each gram of alcohol averages 7.1 calories. The average beer has 13 grams of alcohol—an extra 92.3 calories.				**TOTAL** **1426** CAL

Burn! A Balance of Fitness and Fun

MENU PLANNING NOTES

DEFINITIONS

Flexion:	Decreasing the angle between two bones
Extension:	Increasing the angle between two bones
Dorsiflexion:	Moving the top of the foot toward the shin
Plantarflexion:	Moving the sole of the foot downward
Abduction:	Motion away from the midline
Adduction:	Motion toward the midline
Anterior:	Front portion
Posterior:	Back portion
Lateral:	Outside
Medial::	Inside

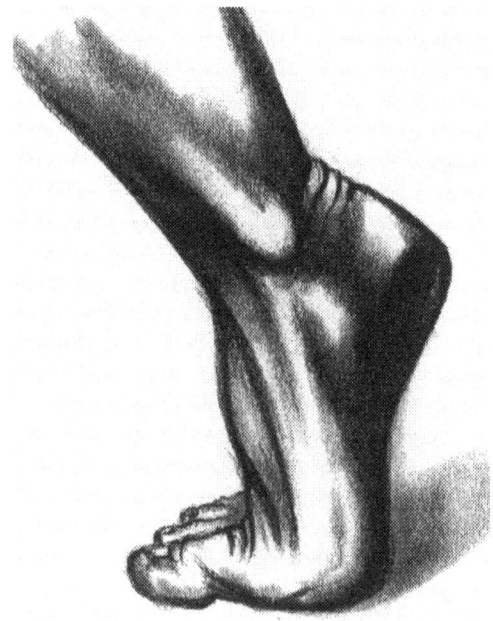

Stretching

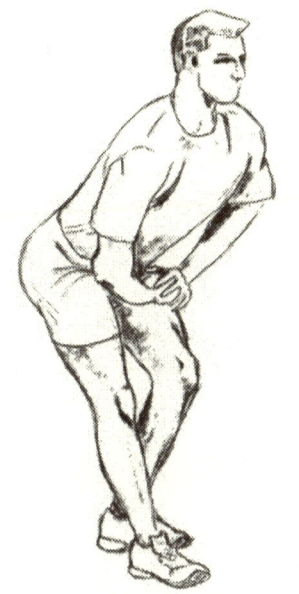

U ntil recently, runners stretched occasion-
ally, at the end of a long run, but rarely
considered it necessary before or during a
run. Increased attention to flexibility has
changed running practice and focused runners
on the value of stretching. Many researchers
believe that careful stretching oxygenates and
hydrates the stretched tissue. Muscles function most effectively in an envi-
ronment of rich blood supply and higher concentrations of oxygen, which
allows proper removal of metabolic byproducts, such as lactic acid. Hydrated
tissue is more flexible and therefore absorbs shock more efficiently, cushioning the concussion that running produces.

You should consider stretching an integral part of your training; but in
order to stretch correctly, you should know a little about your anatomy.

Muscles attach to tendons and tendons, in turn, attach to bones. As we
age, tendons begin to shrink, which puts more pressure on the muscle. All
we can do is counter this natural phenomenon with a few moves of our own.
Stretching elongates these muscles and restores their shape and bounce. It
also helps balance opposing muscle groups, which makes training easier and
more fluid.

Take a look at the diagrams on the following pages to get an idea of what
your muscle groups look like. Note particularly the ones you will be working with as a runner. I have included more muscles than you need to know

as a beginner, but it is interesting to think about what makes your body move. Your new athletic body will be able to extend, flex, and twist. Once you have looked over these detailed illustrations, you will understand my references to the major groups (quadriceps, hamstrings, etc.) as I describe your stretches.

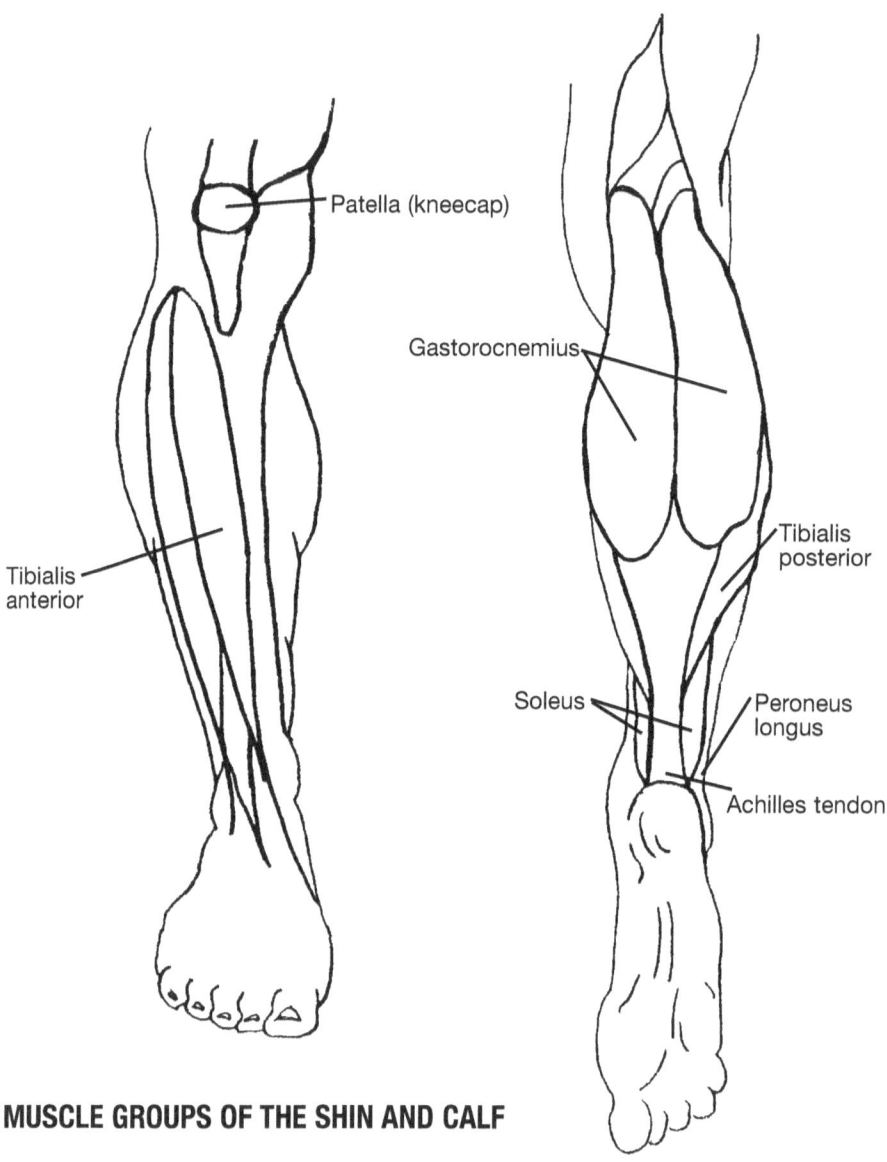

MUSCLE GROUPS OF THE SHIN AND CALF

STRUCTURES OF THE KNEE

Illustrations on this page show the major structures of the knee, including bones, cartilage, muscles, ligaments, and tendons.

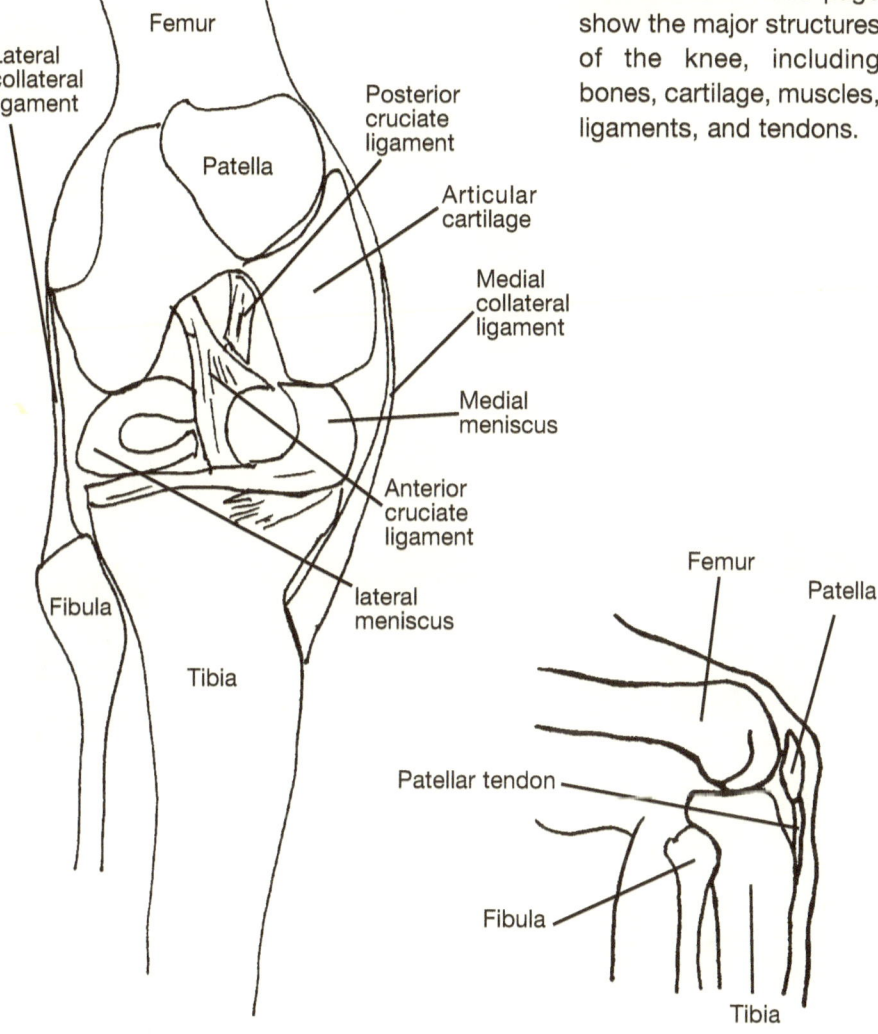

Illustrations on the facing page (46) show the major muscle groups in the shin (lower anterior leg) and the calf (lower posterior leg). *Tibialis anterior* is used for ankle dorsiflexion and foot inversion. *Tibialis posterior* is used for foot inversion and ankle plantarflexion. *Gastrocnemius* produces ankle plantarflexion and knee flexion. *Soleus* is involved with ankle plantarflexion. *Peroneus longus* plantar flexes ankle and helps to support the transverse arch of the foot.

MUSCLE GROUPS OF THE QUADRICEPS, HAMSTRINGS, BUTTOCKS, AND GROIN

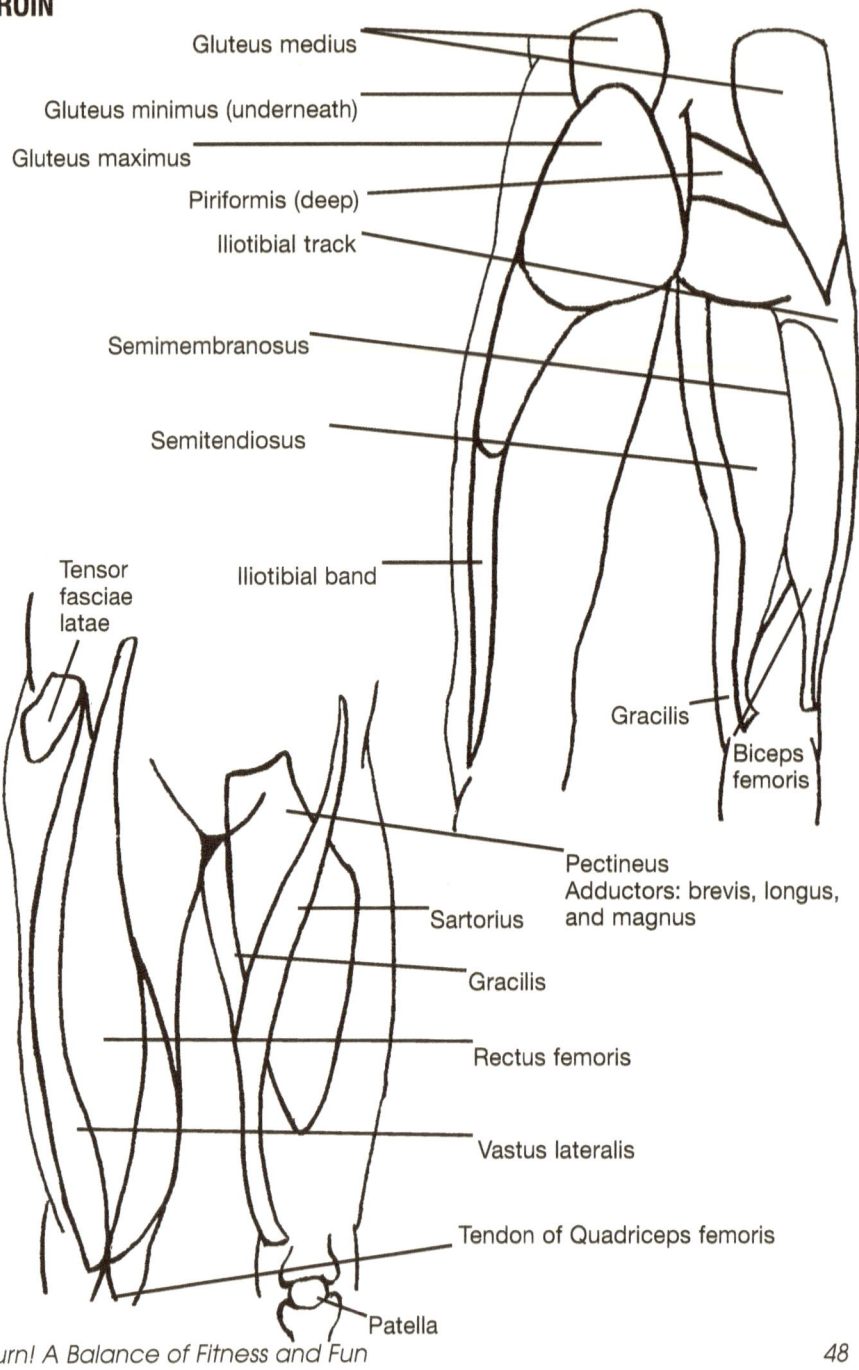

Gluteus medius

Gluteus minimus (underneath)

Gluteus maximus

Piriformis (deep)

Iliotibial track

Semimembranosus

Semitendiosus

Tensor fasciae latae

Iliotibial band

Gracilis

Biceps femoris

Pectineus
Adductors: brevis, longus, and magnus

Sartorius

Gracilis

Rectus femoris

Vastus lateralis

Tendon of Quadriceps femoris

Patella

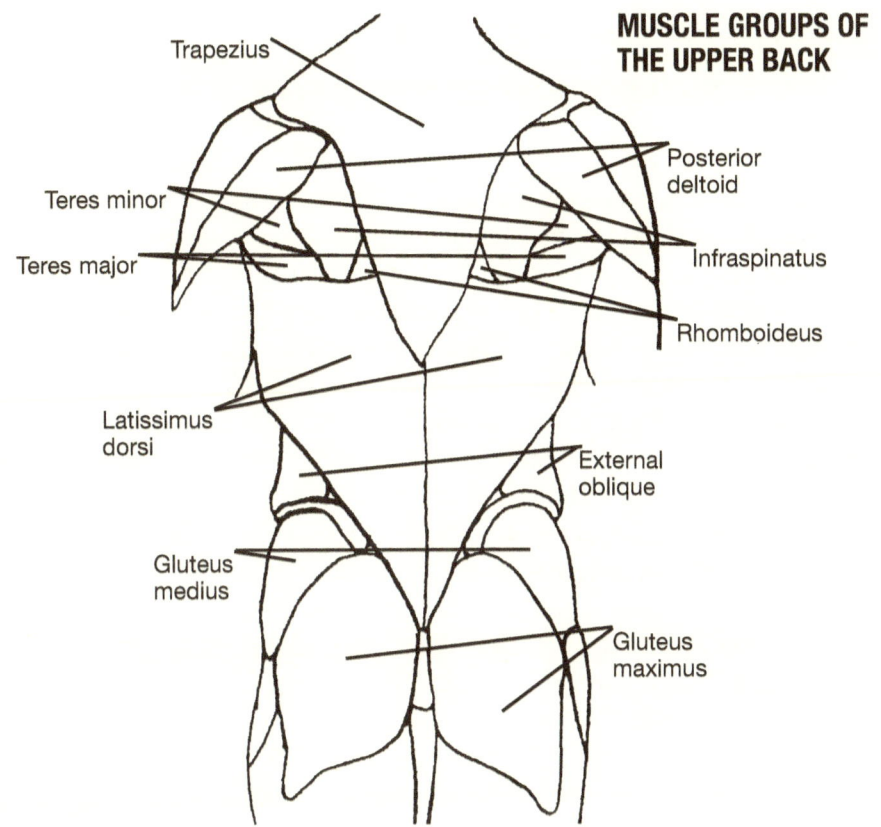

Trapezius

Teres minor

Teres major

Posterior
deltoid

Infraspinatus

Rhomboideus

Latissimus
dorsi

External
oblique

Gluteus
medius

Gluteus
maximus

The illustration above shows muscle systems of the upper back and torso as they relate to the "running muscle" groups of the hips and legs.

Illustrations on the facing page (48) detail the major muscles in the anterior portion of the upper leg (quadriceps), the posterior portion of upper leg (hamstrings), the buttocks (gluteal area) and the groin area. *Piriformis* is a hip rotator. *Rectus femoris, Vastus intermedius, Vastus lateralis,* and *Vastus medialis* extend the leg and knee and flex the hip. *Sartorius* flexes the hip and enables external and internal rotation and knee flexion. *Tensor fascias latae* allows medial rotation, abduction, and maintains tension in the Iliotibial band. *Biceps femoris, Semimembranosus,* and *Semitendinosus* facilitate hip extension and knee flexion. *Gracilis* enables hip adduction and knee flexion. *Gluteus maximus* provides hip extension and lateral rotation, as well as stability to the hip and pelvis. *Gluteus medius* and *minimus* enable hip abduction and medial rotation. *Pectineus, Adductor brevis, Adductor longus, Adductor magnus,* and *Gracilis* facilitate adduction.

STARTING TO STRETCH

During your first few days, just enjoy being outdoors in the fresh air. Walk a little, run a little, and add a few stretches here and there. Join the rest of those folks you have noticed bending trees, holding up buildings, and pushing cars. Stretching will become an important part of your workout—not so much at the start and more concentrated at the conclusion.

Stretching a cold muscle can cause more harm than good and possibly even result in an injury. Warm up a little and get the tightness out. If you do, your stretching session will be more beneficial. Muscles tend to stretch when they are warmed up.

When you begin the stretch, your muscle will contract initially as a defensive mechanism. Breathe again, hold for 5–10 seconds, then continue. The muscle will relax and let you stretch.

Deep breathing brings more oxygen to your cells. This enables the tissues to receive more oxygen so they can lengthen painlessly. Hold for another 25–30 seconds. Ease into the stretch, breathe deeply, and relax and hold. Don't do any bouncing or forcing—just nice, easy stretches that feel very comfortable. Never stretch into pain. Stretch just far enough to feel the tightness, then relax.

Once you start your run, it certainly doesn't hurt to stop once in a while and do some light stretching. Remember you are not racing, just exercising, so get the most out of your workout. Stopping for a light stretch will completely rejuvenate your stride, smoothing out your muscles by elongating them into their normal position—not tight and contracted. This, in turn, brings back your form and makes the rest of your run much easier.

I see people jogging in place while waiting at an intersection or through some other traffic delay. You won't stiffen up doing a 9-minute-per-mile pace. Your time will be better spent doing a few stretches, rather than hopping up and down as if you're looking for the port-a-potty. Just concentrate on the real workers, like the calves, quads, and hamstrings. You'll be more than ready to continue when the light changes to green.

CALF MUSCLES

The calf muscles are important to stretch because of their connection to the knee ligaments at the upper end and to the Achilles tendon at the lower end, around the heel. Tendons don't stretch, so keeping this muscles elongated is critical.

There are two excellent stretches for the calf. The first one is the "curb" stretch. Standing on a curb, or other raised surface, drop your heel down, and let your calf stretch. By standing straight or leaning forward, you can stretch different portions of the calf muscle. Hold the stretch for at least 30 seconds, and then repeat with the other leg. Thirty seconds is a long time, so don't get impatient and cut yourself short.

The other calf stretch is done by standing some distance away from a wall and leaning into it. Varying the distance will stretch different portions of the calf muscle. A straight leg stretches the gastronemius and a bent knee the soleus. Lean forward and put your hands on the wall. Keep the foot of the leg you're stretching flat on the ground, with the leg straight, and bend the other leg as you lean forward. Take a look at the diagram; it will become easier to understand. You should be able to see why varying the distance, and bending the extended knee slightly, will stretch different portions of the muscle. With your leg extended straight back, you will also be stretching your groin at the same time. These stretches are good for preventing both injuries to the Achilles tendon and knee irritation.

STRETCHING THE CALF MUSCLES

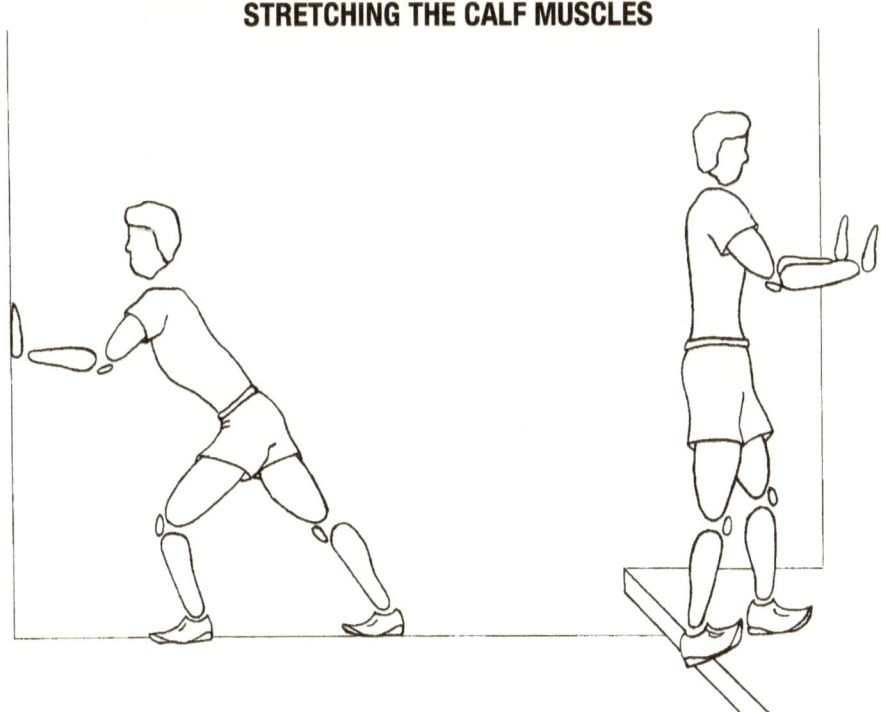

QUADRICEPS

The quadriceps comprise a strong, large muscle group in opposition to the hamstrings. They are relatively easy to stretch. Stand on one leg while you lift the other leg, by holding a foot with the opposite hand. This tends to stretch shin muscles at the same time.

I prefer to stretch by holding one foot with the hand on the same side of the body, for example, left hand holds left foot. Slowly raise the foot up and outward toward your buttocks. This motion is more of an outward swing rather than tucked in toward your buttocks. Hold for at least 30 seconds and repeat with the other leg. If you let your hand slide more toward the toes on the foot you are holding, you will also stretch the shin area.

As with the other muscle groups, this muscle is much easier to stretch after being warmed up. It feels good to stretch during a run, and stretching properly will definitely restore the bounce and spring to your stride.

STRETCHING THE QUADRICEPS

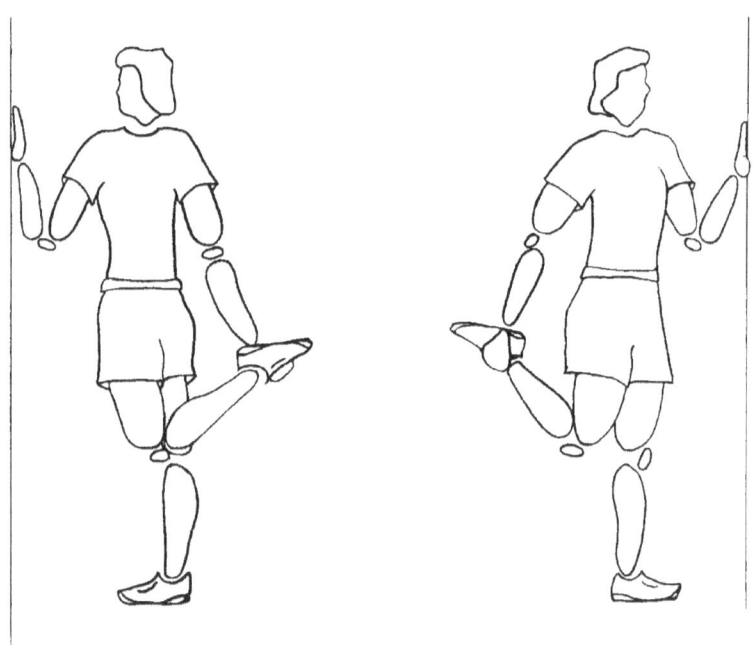

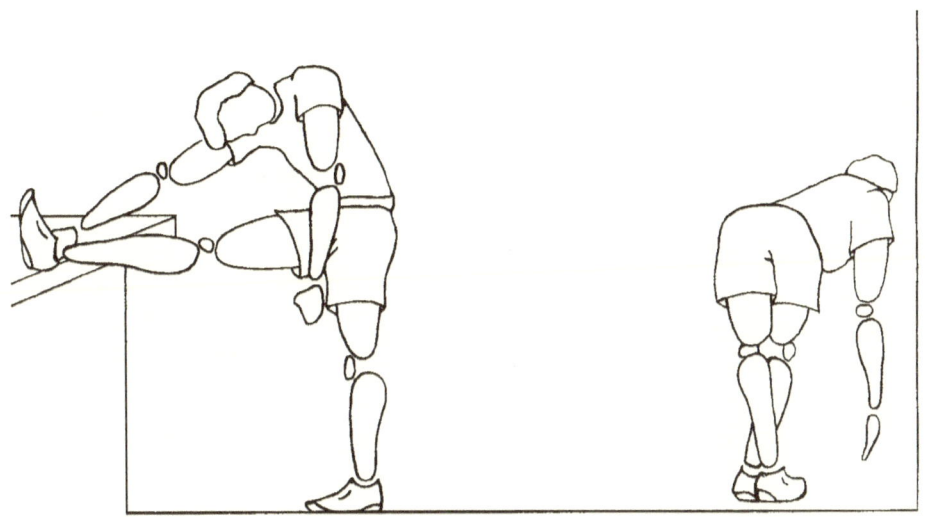

HAMSTRINGS

Placing your heel on an elevated surface easily stretches the hamstrings. Don't pick a surface too high—just elevated enough to be comfortable. Once you have your foot up in the air, lean forward and touch your toes, or just lean forward until you feel the stretch.

Easy does it. Don't over-stretch, just enough to feel the tug in your hamstring. Don't strain your back on this stretch either. Lean forward just enough to feel the back of your leg being stretched. At the beginning of a run you might alter this stretch by extending one leg out in front of the other, not elevated but in front. Bend the weight-bearing leg while keeping the extended leg straight.

After your run, try another good hamstrings stretch: Lie on your back, clasp your knee to your chest, and hold for 30 seconds. Touching your toes, or attempting to touch your toes, is also a useful stretch for your hamstrings, lower back, piriformis, and glutes. Alternating one leg crossed over the other while you touch your toes will stretch piriformis and glutes even more. Refer to the illustration.

GLUTEAL AREA

Many of these muscles will be stretched while you are stretching your hamstrings. There are a couple of extra stretches that isolate the gluteus maximus, medius, minimus, and piriformis a little more.

Sitting on the ground, raise one leg over the other by bending the knee. Now move, in this case, the right knee to the left and hold. This really stretches the piriformis. Raising both knees toward your chest, while lying on the ground, will also stretch the glutes and lower back.

ILIOTIBIAL BAND

The iliotibial is a thick band of fibrous tissue that begins in the hip region and is sometimes considered an extension of the tensor fascia latae muscle, which gives it tension. The iliotibial band holds the leg straight and gives the thigh muscle a chance to relax. It extends down the outside of the leg and then crosses over to connect to the shinbone just below the knee. Where it passes the knee area, small bursae prevent it from rubbing against the knee bone. Stretching helps keep these areas from getting inflamed.

The best iliotibial stretch is to hold your arms above your head with your legs crossed, one foot behind the other and lean to the side of your rear foot. Alternate rear foot and stretch the other side.

GROIN

Your adductor muscles are located in the inner thigh area of your upper leg and groin. These muscles should be stretched frequently to avoid a groin pull. Groin injuries take a long time to heal, so don't ignore these stretches.

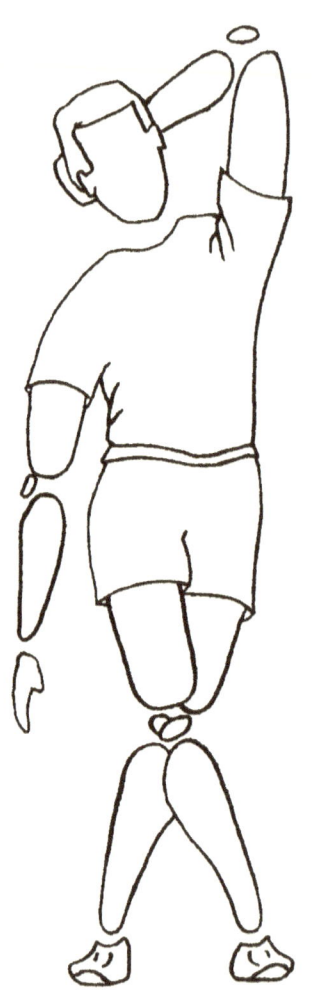

STRETCHING THE ILIOTIBIAL BAND

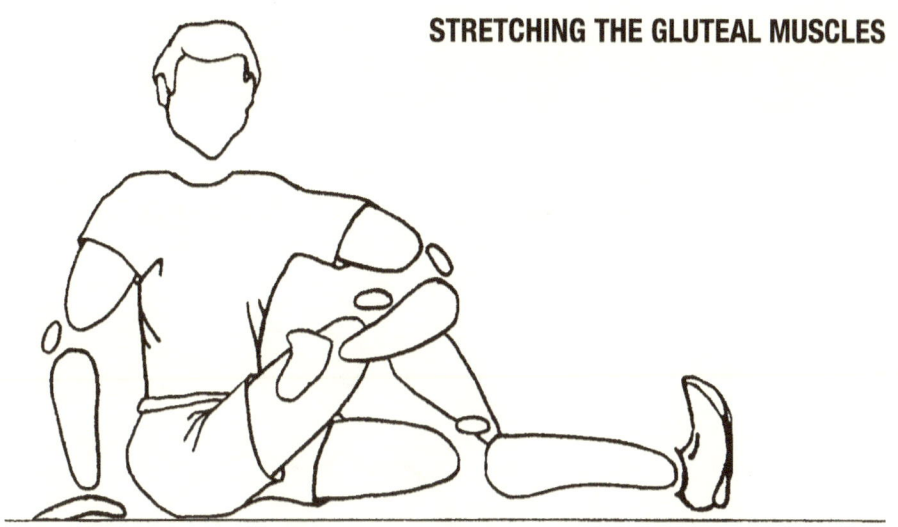

STRETCHING THE GLUTEAL MUSCLES

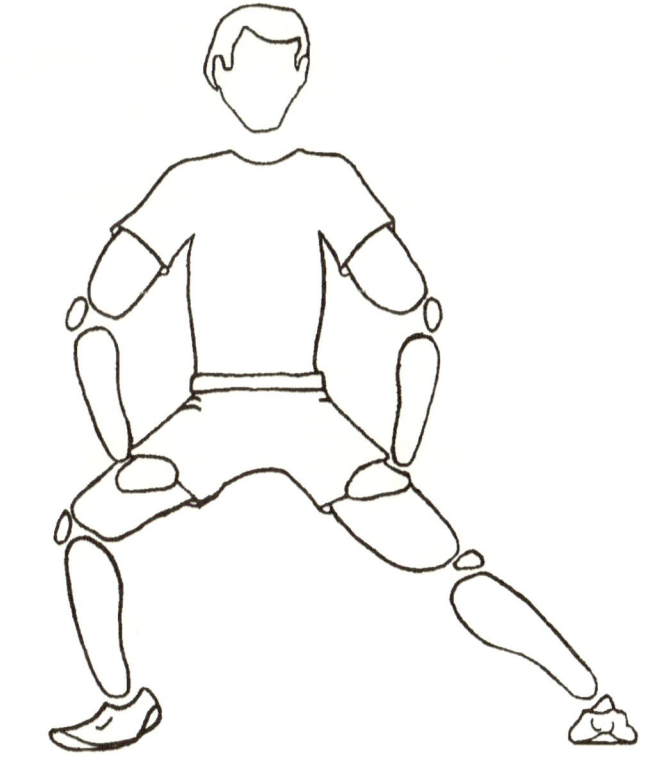

STRETCHING THE ADDUCTOR MUSCLES

Stretching

The inner thigh stretch is similar to the hamstring stretch, except you are facing 90 degrees to the left or right. Put your foot on a raised surface and lean sideways until you feel the stretch.

The next one is simple: you just spread your legs and lean from side to side by bending one knee at a time. Before you sit down, try some squats for stretches of your groin, Achilles tendon and back. Try to keep your heels flat on the ground.

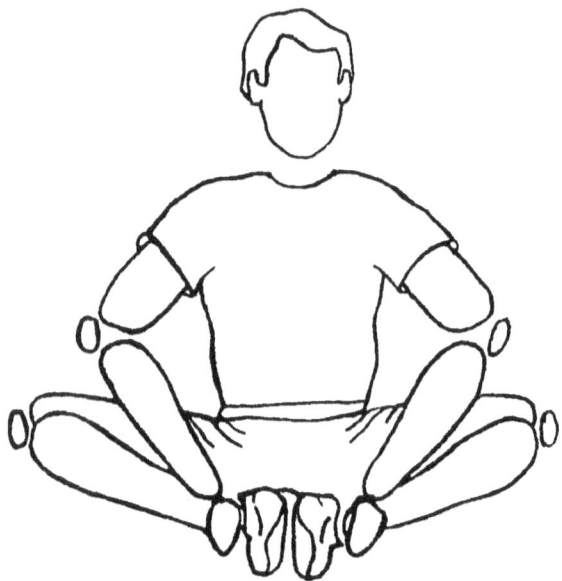

THE BUTTERFLY

The next two are done from a sitting position. Extend your legs in front of you and twist them so your toes turn inward. Last is the butterfly. Pull your feet in toward your groin while letting your knees drop to the sides. Easy does it; breathe deeply.

NECK AND BACK

Stretching your neck and back will help you relax and prevent that "uptight" feeling. You don't want your shoulders to be flexed and bunched up. When you relax your shoulders and back, the rest of your body seems to follow. Your arms tend to drop down lower, where they should be. Just think about running relaxed—with everything in line. "Running tall" is a good description of what you want to achieve.

The stretch you used for your hamstrings will also produce good results for your back. For your neck, just roll your head around, back and forth

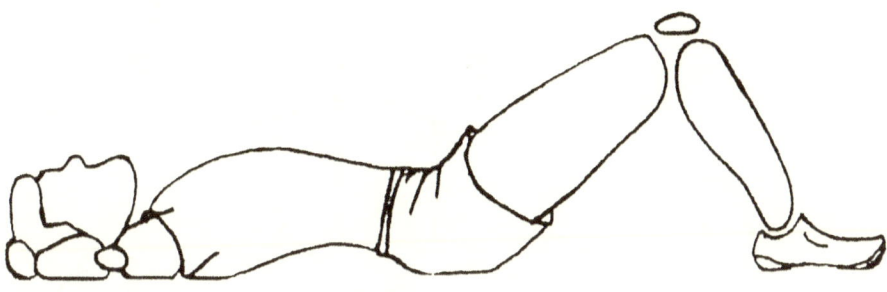

STRETCHING THE NECK AND BACK

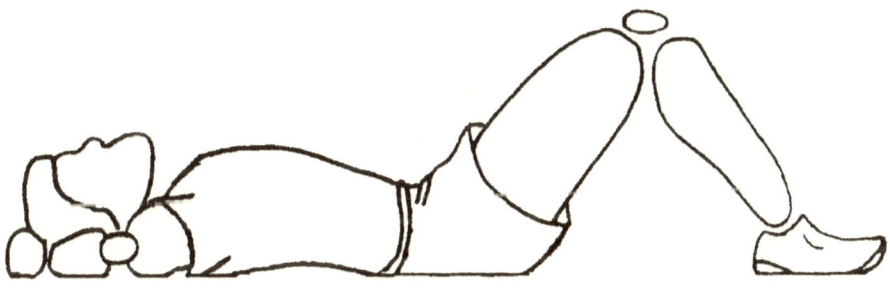

While you are still on the ground, lie on your back, placing the soles of your feet on the ground. Breathe out and drop your lower back to the ground.

Roll over and get on your hands and knees, then press your belly toward the ground and your head and buttocks toward the sky. Now reverse it. Extend your back toward the sky and drop your head and buttocks to the ground.

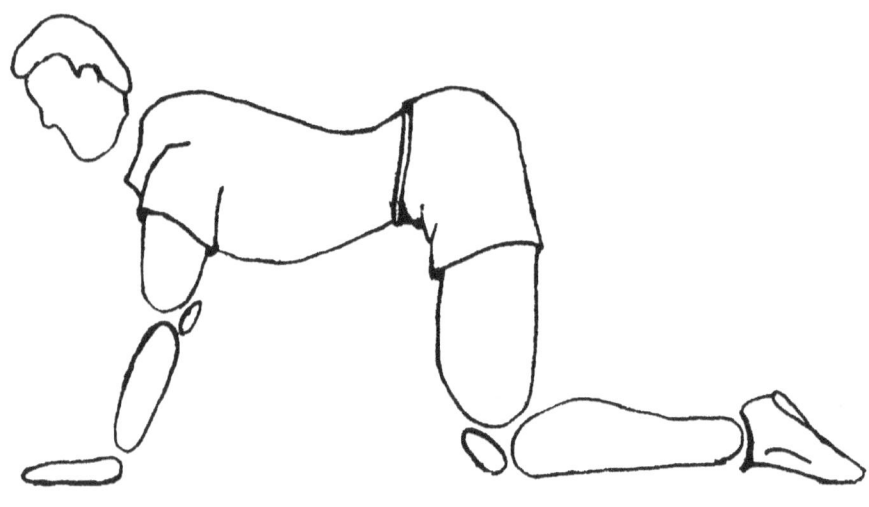

STRETCHING YOUR LOWER BACK

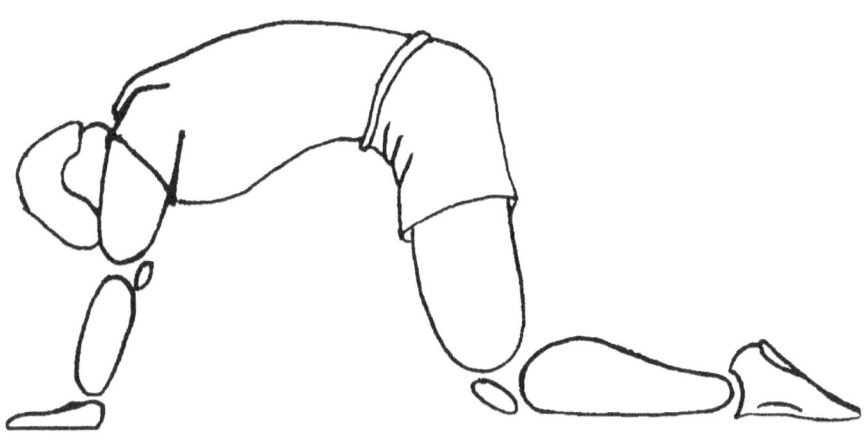

These stretches should be sufficient to get you started and help you during your run, even while waiting for red lights. At the conclusion of your run, you should add a few more stretches that we haven't covered.

Your lower back is one of the areas that should get a little stretching at the beginning while you are stretching the other muscle groups. Concentrate a little extra time on isolating the lower back completely.

Leaning forward and backward will get you started loosening up your lower back. Don't do any bouncing on the forward lean. If you can't touch your toes, don't force it; just stretch until you are comfortable. Crossing one leg in front of the other while you lean forward will also stretch your hamstrings while you work on your back. Hip twists are simple and easy to perform while you cool down. Just put your hands on your hips and twist your torso—left, right, and hold.

You are probably tired, so finish these stretches on the ground—if you are fortunate enough to have some grass available. Legs straight out in front, lean forward and attempt to touch your toes. No bouncing. Now get comfortable and lie down on your back. Lift one knee to your chest, hold with your hands, and alternate. This one is great for back and quads. Another good stretch for your lower back is to cross one leg over the other and keep it straight and extended to the side. Now try to get up.

Just kidding—but it is a comfortable position on a sunny day.

Consistent stretching at the conclusion of your run will help to prevent muscle soreness and injury, preparing you for your next workout. Besides feeling good, stretching contributes to better joint function, increases production of synovial fluid (joint lube), improves circulation, and, of course, increases flexibility. The main thing to remember is that if you don't take the time to stretch, you may end up with an injury that could have been prevented. Stretching should always be the silent, but absolutely necessary, part of your training. It's easy to skip the stretching when you are pressed for time, but wiser to shorten your run and add more speed.

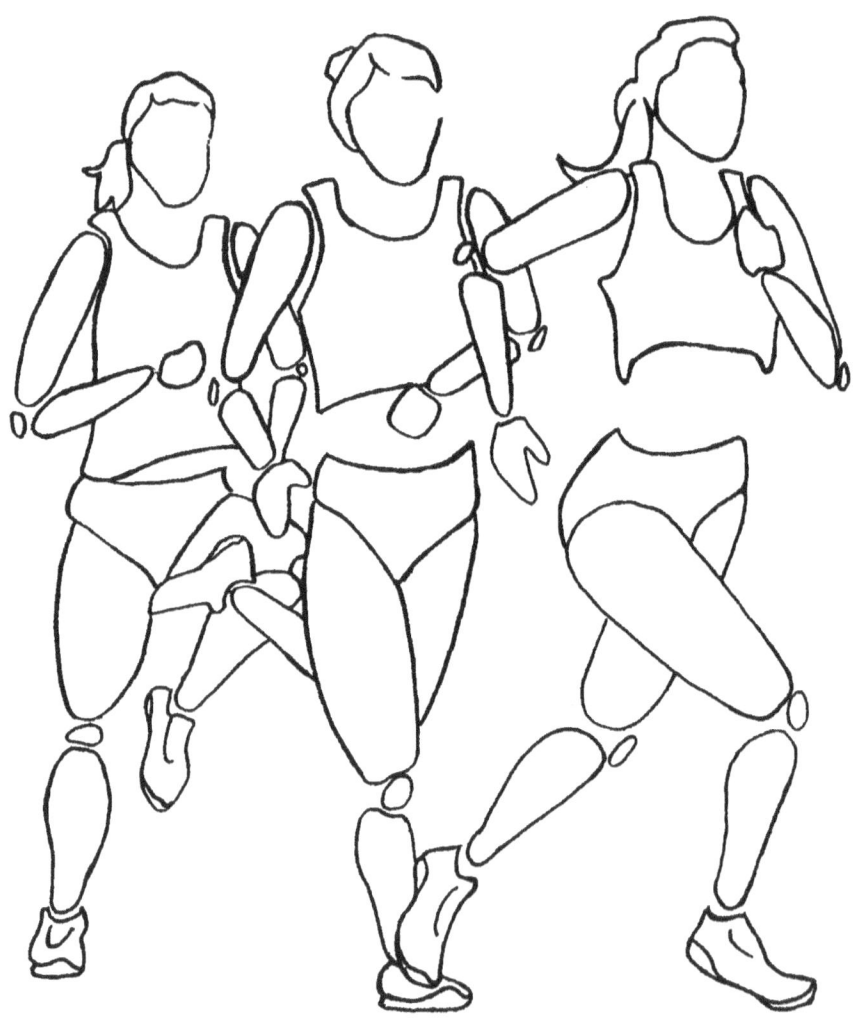

Training

You can start this program walking, running or doing a combination of both. The main training schedule will take you from a walking start all the way to serious runner in 16 weeks.

This schedule demands the ultimate commitment. I've included three other training regimens that require somewhat less commitment. No matter which one you choose, you will have to stay with it and plan to "burn" those calories. Just follow the times—and later the mileage—as you become more physically conditioned.

This is your program; you can increase or decrease at your own pace. It's just like a 5K race—set the tempo that suits you, but get the job done. The main point to remember is you have to "burn" to lose weight. You have to work hard to get the results you want. An easy jog in the park may be nice for an off day, but the workout day has to be worthwhile. You have to sweat and pant to make it count. How do you like it so far?

The main schedule is interspersed with many helpful training hints. In the three other schedules, these hints are omitted, so you might scan the main schedule before beginning your training.

No matter which schedule you start with, pick a time of day for training that best suits your particular lifestyle. You don't want to feel rushed or pressed for time. The morning is usually a good choice because it sets up the rest of the day. After a good workout, you will be relaxed and ready to take on the activities and challenges of the day. Even your meals tend to fall into place better with a morning workout. You can have a nice breakfast or lunch, depending on how early you trained, without being concerned about running on a full stomach later in the day.

Afternoon training sometimes gets pushed around because of the day's commitments and ends up being rushed and not as pleasant as it should be. Evening training will conflict with your dinner. Running before dinner will make your dinner late and if you wait until after dinner you will be getting close to bedtime and might get too wound up to sleep restfully.

Now that you have decided on a time of day, it's important to pick a nice location to start your program. It may be necessary to drive to a park or bike trail in a nice river setting. It's worth the trek because your mood is a very important segment of your overall training. Are you ready? Let's go "burnnnnn."

MAIN SCHEDULE

WEEK 1

Monday	Tuesday	Wednesday	Thursday	Friday	Saturday	Sunday	Total Time
20–25	20–25	20–25	rest	20–25	20–25	rest	1:40–2:05

NOTE: Watch your posture. Swing your arms straight—forward and backward, not side to side. Keep your hands relaxed, no fists. As you pick up the pace you should continue to increase the time a little more so that your second week will look like this:

Monday	Tuesday	Wednesday	Thursday	Friday	Saturday	Sunday	Total Time
25–30	25–30	25–30	rest	25–30	25–30	rest	2:05–2:30

WEEK 2

NOTE: How do the shoes feel? Keep stretching. Drink plenty of water.

You are now walking 25–30 minutes a day, five times a week, and you should be feeling pretty comfortable with your schedule. Most of you will want to stay at this pace for another week or two. For those of you who feel you are ready for the next step, it is time to increase the pace. The best way to do this is to go over to a nearby campus with a track.

Try to utilize the outside lanes during your regular workouts. Normally, the inner lanes will be used for serious training and track meets. Every once in a while, slip into the inner lane for a lap—just to check your pace.

You don't want to get in the way of school activities or serious training in progress, so pick a time when the track is free. In order to record your speed accurately, you'll have to use the inside lane. Each lap is equal to 1/4 of a mile (400 meters or 440 yards), so four laps will equal one mile.

Start your clock and walk at a good steady pace, a little quicker than your beginning pace during the previous week, for one lap, and check your time. For example, four minutes will equate to a 16-minute mile. Don't stop walking, but continue on for one and a half miles, which will be six laps. For those of you starting this program in the winter, with two feet of snow outside, you will have to accomplish this on a treadmill. To do this, walk or run for one mile and note the time it took to complete. That is your pace per mile. Divide that time by four and you will have your lap time. For example, after one mile of walking you noted your time was 20 minutes. Divide by four and your lap time is five minutes. If you are running and your time is 10 minutes at the one-mile point, that works out to 2-1/2-minute laps.

For the next couple of weeks, don't worry about the distance, just try to work up to 40–45 minutes at your new, timed pace. Most of you are going to want to go back to your trail along the river or quiet neighborhood park. You will only be using the track once in awhile to check your progress and pace. Later on in your training, you may use the track for timed laps to pick up your pace and endurance.

WEEK 3

Monday	Tuesday	Wednesday	Thursday	Friday	Saturday	Sunday	Total Time
30–35	30–35	30–35	rest	30–35	30–35	rest	2:30–2:55

WEEK 4

Monday	Tuesday	Wednesday	Thursday	Friday	Saturday	Sunday	Total Time
35–40	35–40	35–40	rest	35–40	35–40	rest	2:55–3:20

NOTE: Check your form. Run tall. Drinking lots of water. Keep stretching. Lower your arms.

WEEK 5

Monday	Tuesday	Wednesday	Thursday	Friday	Saturday	Sunday	Total Time/ Miles
40–45	40–45	40–45	rest	40–45	40–45	rest	3–4 hours/ 12–15 miles

NOTE: Avoid too much, too soon. Follow the 10% rule: increase your mileage by no more than 10% per week. Keep your log updated. Check your stride.

For simplicity, let's say our new pace is 15 minutes per mile. At that pace, you are covering three miles in a 45-minute workout. Five days a week will give you a total weekly mileage of 15 miles. It's time to add some running.

Up until this point you haven't really started to sweat—maybe just a little perspiration. Now we should move into some slow "burning." Make sure you are drinking your water. It is very important to replenish any water you lose during exercise. The more water you can drink, the less water your body has to store. Sports drinks are also considered an excellent method of replenishing your liquid loss.

Before getting too far along in your new running/walking program, take the time to analyze your new running shoes. How do they feel? You may want to experiment with the way you lace the shoes or the tightness. Just small changes, nothing major, unless your shoes are really bothering you.

Make sure the rest of your clothes feel all right and are completely comfortable and appropriate. For instance, running in cold weather will take a little more planning than a fun run in the sun. How chilly it becomes will dictate how much clothing to put on, but keep in mind, your body will be warming up by the first mile and you may have over dressed. For temperatures ranging from 35 degrees Fahrenheit to 50 degrees Fahrenheit, I suggest a long-sleeved t-shirt and lightweight jacket, along with warm-up pants. Hats and gloves are also a must, to keep the heat in and extremities warm. Make sure the clothing you wear breathes well; otherwise you will perspire too much. You'll be soaking wet and you will dehydrate much quicker. The jacket, being lightweight, can be removed when you warm up and tied around your waist.

Wind is another consideration. Wind will lower the temperature a few degrees and, obviously, the harder it blows, the colder it becomes. Try to run into the wind at the beginning of your run, so that by the time you turn around for your return, you will have the wind at your back. Running into the wind when you are warm and sweaty is uncomfortable on a cold and blustery day.

In areas where it snows and the temperatures drop below freezing, footing becomes an important factor. Light snow on a dry surface is usually pretty safe. You can navigate reasonably well and have a good time. Avoid running on frozen surfaces where there are large areas of continuous ice. Slipping and falling on the ice can be extremely dangerous and excruciatingly painful. The slip seems to accelerate the fall, so it becomes more like a slam-dunk. Stay off the ice!

In the fall, be careful running on trails and bike paths in areas where leaves have shed after their last blast of brilliance. The leaves tend to hide objects like rocks, roots, and uneven cracks in the path that normally would be noticed and avoided. Enjoy these areas at a more leisurely walking pace, which will allow you to keep your footing and absorb the beauty of the changing fall colors. Later, you'll be ready for a refreshing run outside the woods.

I should take the time here to mention some tips for running the streets and highways. First of all, avoid highways at all costs if you possibly can. The only reason to run next to a highway would be in order to be seen—and who cares? Everybody has seen runners, so get off the highway and back on quiet, parallel streets. Avoid streets with a large camber. For drainage, some streets are sloped from the middle toward the curb. This camber is tough on runners, similar to running on a sloped beach, and may cause problems with your foot plant and possibly minor injuries.

I prefer to run against the traffic—just so I can see what the drivers are up to. Be extremely cautious. Look for cars making a right turn onto your street. The drivers will tend to have all their attention looking left and down the street for merging traffic and will not notice you approaching from their right.

Try to keep your running surface soft—the softer the better. Cement is the worst. It doesn't give at all. If you have to pick a surface that is paved, try to stick with asphalt. Trails are great when they are smooth and hard packed. Roots and rocks tend to spoil some would-be great trails. Bark on city trails can cause uneven footing; such trails are better suited for walking. The beach is great if you can time it to arrive at extremely low tide. This will give you an even, hard-packed surface. Otherwise you will be running on a slant, similar to roads with camber discussed above, which is definitely not good, or in the soft sand, which extremely uncomfortable and could cause shin splints. I will discuss injuries later.

Now that we you have added the running, continue to stay with the 40–45 minutes workout, putting in as much running as you can during that period. Concentrate on your form. Keep your body straight. Don't lean forward. Make sure you land on your heel and push off with the ball of your foot.

WEEK 6

Monday	Tuesday	Wednesday	Thursday	Friday	Saturday	Sunday	Total Time/ Miles
40–45 / 3.5–4.0	40–45 / 3.5–4.0	40–45 / 3.5–4.0	rest	40–45 / 3.5–4.0	40–45 / 3.5–4.0	rest	3–4 hours / 17.5–20 miles

NOTE: Are you getting your rest and a good night's sleep? Drink lots of water. Stretch. Keep up your log.

WEEKS 7–9

Continue with this program until you can complete the entire 45-minute session running, with maybe a couple of stops for stretching. You may feel that you have reached a point in your training where you are achieving good results. This may be a good place to level off for a while.

For those of you moving on, it's time to head back to the track to recheck your pace. Remember, one lap is equal to 1/4 of a mile; so four laps will be one mile. Let's say your lap takes 2-1/2 minutes and you continue at that same pace for one mile. That would equate to a 10-minute mile. In other words, it takes you 10 minutes to run one mile. Easy. A 2-minute lap would be an 8-minute mile and so on. Now with this little bit of knowledge, it will be easier to switch your training program from time to miles. For example, if you want to run five miles at a nine-minute-per-mile pace, it should take you 45 minutes. This tells you right where you are in your training.

Adding some more mileage will take a couple of weeks. The standard formula for adding mileage, and at the same time trying to avoid injuries, is to increase mileage by only 10% per week.

To do this, we will rearrange your schedule to include one day of track work or speed work on the road and we will designate one day as your long run. The long run day will be the day we will continue to add the mileage—until we arrive at 30 miles per week. At this point (Week 10), you are only five miles away from reaching that goal, so we can push it up slowly over the next few weeks and you will be at 29 miles per week in Week 12.

WEEK 10

Monday	Tuesday	Wednesday	Thursday	Friday	Saturday	Sunday	Total Miles
5 miles	track 3.5 miles	5 miles	rest	5 miles	6.5 miles	rest	25 miles

WEEK 11

Monday	Tuesday	Wednesday	Thursday	Friday	Saturday	Sunday	Total Miles
5 miles	track 4.5 miles	5 miles	rest	5 miles	7.5 miles	rest	27 miles

WEEK 12

Monday	Tuesday	Wednesday	Thursday	Friday	Saturday	Sunday	Total Miles
5 miles	track 5 miles	5 miles	rest	5 miles	9 miles	rest	29 miles

Twenty-nine miles a week is a laudable accomplishment. If you reach this goal in 12 weeks, you will have accomplished a great milestone in your new life. For most of you, this can be considered a plateau in your program. By readjusting your training days, you can create your own program that could better suit your present goals and needs.

You might feel that five days a week is preventing you from accomplishing some other goals—or putting too many time constraints on an already strained weekly schedule. You can add another rest day and pick up the mileage on the remaining four days.

Monday	Tuesday	Wednesday	Thursday	Friday	Saturday	Sunday	Total Miles
track 5 miles	7 miles	rest	7 miles	rest	10 miles	rest	29 miles

NOTE: Running burns 100 calories/mile. To lose 1 pound = 3600 calories or 36 miles. Do you need a smaller size in your running shorts?

Take a couple of weeks to make this change and you might feel much more comfortable.

TRACK DAY
- 1 mile warm-up—1 minute rest between laps
- 4x440 timed
- 1 mile timed
- 4x440 timed
- 1 mile cool down—total 5 miles

If you want to round your program off at 30 miles a week, you can add an extra mile to your long run on Saturday and make it 11 miles.

Training on the track once a week shouldn't be considered punishment but an opportunity to increase your pace and help build up more stamina.

Some people just don't like the track. I can remember when I was in high school being told to run a lap as a form of punishment for goofing off. Maybe you had the same experience and still associate running laps with bad behavior.

Working on your speed doesn't have to be done on the track. Many runners prefer to incorporate their speed work into normal runs on the road.

Once you have warmed up for a mile and done some mild stretching, it's time to pick up the pace a little. Pick out a landmark a few blocks away, increase your pace, and hold it until you reach that mark. Slow back to your normal pace and repeat this scenario several times during your run. This is often referred to as "fartlek" or fun running. It does put a little extra boost into your road running and it leaves you with a feeling of accomplishment.

As you push the pace, you should be aware of physical changes that may take place. Normal exercise is considered "aerobic." When you exercise, you draw in oxygen through your lungs to fuel your muscles. Once you start to push your body past being comfortable, you will eventually start to run out of oxygen to fuel your muscles. Your lungs can only supply a certain amount for demand. At that point, you start operating "anaerobically," or without air. You have reached your anaerobic threshold and pretty soon you will be though running. In this stage, your muscles will start burning stored glycogen for energy. The byproduct of anaerobic training is called lactic acid or oxygen debt. This will leave your muscles sore and require some rest to recover before resuming your training program.

Now you can move up to some really serious "burning." Be cautious any time you begin a new program, run a different course, or especially run on a different surface. Starting a workout with hills can cause some problems if you don't work into it slowly. The most common injury, as a result of running downhill, is shin splints. Even long continuous grades can cause a problem. Your first session should consist of short, not-too-steep hills. Each week, as you feel more comfortable, you can increase the intensity.

Hill running will require a little different posture, so that you stay smooth and efficient. Running uphill, obviously, is going to require more energy and stamina. Pump your arms more than you normally do on the flat surfaces. Shorten your stride a little to accommodate the degree of incline. Don't lean forward; try to stay straight. Coming back down the hill, gravity is on your side; but don't let that make you overstrike because you will pound your quadriceps and hamstrings. Keep the stride comfortable and try to glide down the hill. Keep your posture straight and don't lean back. Let your arms drop down a little lower in a more relaxed position.

With this kind of a workout week, you should probably be back on a five-day schedule.

Monday	Tuesday	Wednesday	Thursday	Friday	Saturday	Sunday	Total Miles
5 miles slow	5 miles track	rest	5 miles slow	5 miles hills	rest	10 miles	30 miles

NOTE: How do your shins feel? Be careful on those hills.

You may want to stay at this level for a while. This is probably the best overall workout you will need. It includes one day of speed work, either on the track or the roads, one day of hill repeats, and one long run. The other days are easy and you still have two rest days.

To train for longer races, you will have to step up the intensity a little and add some more mileage. Make sure you stick with the 10% rule, as you add mileage. Right now that would be no more than three more miles per week. Keep your track day and hill day at five miles each and add to the other days.

WEEK 13

Monday	Tuesday	Wednesday	Thursday	Friday	Saturday	Sunday	Total Miles
6 miles easy	5 miles track	rest	5 miles hills	6 miles easy	rest	11 miles long, slow	33 miles

WEEK 14

Monday	Tuesday	Wednesday	Thursday	Friday	Saturday	Sunday	Total Miles
7 miles	5 miles track	rest	5 miles hills	7 miles easy	rest	12 miles long, slow	36 miles

WEEK 15

Monday	Tuesday	Wednesday	Thursday	Friday	Saturday	Sunday	Total Miles
8 miles	5 miles	rest	5 miles hills	8 miles easy	rest	13 miles	39 miles

WEEK 16

Monday	Tuesday	Wednesday	Thursday	Friday	Saturday	Sunday	Total Miles
8 miles	5 miles	rest	5 miles hills	8 miles easy	rest	14 miles	40 miles

To get your mileage above 40, you can continue to add to your easy days—up to 10 miles a day—or add some more to your long run. If you add to your long run, you might want to switch your off day to Sunday.

Monday	Tuesday	Wednesday	Thursday	Friday	Saturday	Sunday	Total Miles
8 miles	5 miles	rest	5 miles hills	8 miles easy	rest	18 miles	44 miles

Changing from two days off to one day off would look like this:

Monday	Tuesday	Wednesday	Thursday	Friday	Saturday	Sunday	Total Miles
5–8 miles easy	5 miles	5–7 miles track	6–7 miles easy	5–8 miles hills	rest	12–15 miles	38–50 miles

To improve, you have to either run faster or farther—or better yet, a combination of both. Your speed work can be done on the track or the roads. You can even alternate every other week to the track and get some good tempo running on the roads the following week.

Another day should be used for hill training or hill sprints. This will really build your stamina and strength. Remember to keep your form good up and down the hills.

When you do use the track, try to get your warm-up and cool-down miles around the school instead of adding more laps to your routine. This will generally set you up for a good run by getting you relaxed and putting your mind in a gentle state. Of course, the cool-down mile will also be enjoyable because you have just completed a good workout. Now you can enjoy the surroundings as you cool down.

WALKING SCHEDULE

All times are given in hours and minutes.

Week	Monday	Tuesday	Wednesday	Thursday	Friday	Saturday	Sunday	Time
1.	20–25	20–25	20–25	rest	20–25	20–25	rest	1:40–2:05
2.	Repeat week 1.							
3.	25–30	25–30	25–30	rest	25–30	25–30	rest	2:05–2:30
4.	Repeat week 3.							
5.	30–35	30–35	30–35	rest	30–35	30–35	rest	2:30–2:55
6.	Repeat week 5.							
7.	35–40	35–40	35–40	rest	35–40	35–40	rest	2:55–3:20
8.	Repeat week 7.							
9.	40–45	40–45	40–45	rest	40–45	40–45	rest	3:20–3:45
10.	Repeat week 9.							

NOTE: You are much stronger now and feeling more physically fit. To add a little more challenge to your workout, you may want to try walking up and down hills once or twice a week. Not only will this add more stamina to your conditioning, it will train you for new vistas on mountain trails.

Week	Monday	Tuesday	Wednesday	Thursday	Friday	Saturday	Sunday	Time
11.	45–50	45–50	45–50	rest	45–50	45–50	rest	3:45–4:10
12.	Repeat week 11.							
13.	50–55	50–55	50–55	rest	50–55	50–55	rest	4:10–4:35
14.	Repeat week 13.							
15.	55–60	55–60	55–60	rest	55–60	55–60	rest	4:35–5:00
16.	Repeat week 15.							

Four months later, you are walking approximately 20 miles a week and feeling good. Depending on how comfortable you are with your walking program, you may want to consider adding some running to your schedule. If you do, take it easy and just add a little at a time. Refer to Week 6 on the main schedule.

WALK-RUN SCHEDULE

If you have already been running and walking a little, you can start around Week 6 on the main schedule. Refer to the more detailed program on page 74.

Week	Monday	Tuesday	Wednesday	Thursday	Friday	Saturday	Sunday	Time/ Miles
1.	40–45 minutes 3.5–4.0 miles	40–45 minutes 3.5–4.0 miles	40–45 minutes 3.5–4.0 miles	rest	40–45 minutes 3.5–4.0 miles	40–45 minutes 3.5–4.0 miles	rest	3:20–3:45/ 17.5–20 miles
2.	Repeat week 1.							
3.	Repeat week 2.							
4.	Repeat week 3.							
5.	Repeat week 4.							
6.	4–5 miles	4–5 miles	4–5 miles	rest	4–5 miles	4–5 miles	rest	20–25 miles
						Note: Begin all running.		
7.	Repeat week 6.							
8.	Repeat week 7.							
9.	5 miles	4.5 miles track	5 miles	rest	5 miles	6.5 miles	rest	26 miles
				Note: Add some speed work once a week.				
10.	Repeat week 9.							
11.	5 miles	4.5 miles track	5 miles	rest	5 miles	7.5 miles	rest	27 miles
12.	Repeat week 11.							
13.	5 miles	5 miles track	5 miles	rest	5 miles	9 miles	rest	29 miles
14.	Repeat week 13.							
15.	5 miles	5 miles track	rest	10 miles	5 miles easy	5 miles hills	rest	30 miles
			Note: Change rest day and add hills on Saturday.					
16.	Repeat week 15.							

RUNNING SCHEDULE

If you are already a seasoned runner, you will probably choose to start around Week 10 on the main schedule.

Week	Monday	Tuesday	Wednesday	Thursday	Friday	Saturday	Sunday	Miles
1.	5 miles	3.5 miles track	5 miles	rest	5 miles	6.5 miles	rest	25 miles
2.	Repeat week 1.							
3.	5 miles	4 miles track	5 miles	rest	5 miles	7 miles	rest	26 miles
4.	Repeat week 3.							
5.	5 miles	4.5 miles track	5 miles	rest	5 miles	8 miles	rest	27 miles
6.	Repeat week 5.							
7.	5 miles	5 miles track	5 miles	rest	5 miles	8 miles	rest	28 miles
8.	Repeat week 7.							
9.	5 miles	5 miles track	5 miles	rest	5 miles	9 miles	rest	29 miles
10.	6 miles	5 miles track	5 miles	rest	5 miles	10 miles	rest	31 miles
11.	7 miles	5 miles track	5 miles	rest	5 miles	11 miles	rest	33 miles
12.	8 miles	5 miles track	5 miles	rest	5 miles	12 miles	rest	35 miles
13.	8 miles	5 miles track	5 miles	rest	5 miles	13 miles	rest	36 miles
14.	9 miles	5 miles track	5 miles	rest	5 miles	14 miles	rest	38 miles
15.	9 miles	5 miles track	5 miles	rest	5 miles	15 miles	rest	39 miles
16.	10 miles	5 miles track	5 miles	rest	5 miles	15 miles	rest	40 miles

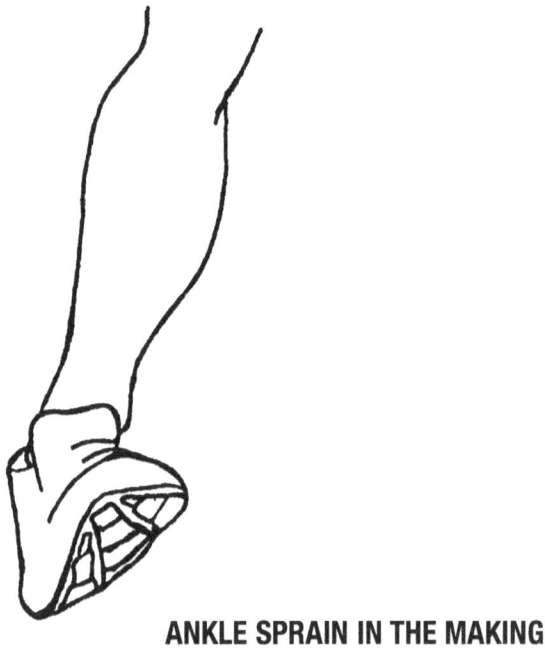

ANKLE SPRAIN IN THE MAKING

Injuries

Unfortunately, this chapter had to be included. If you are extremely fortunate, you may be able to skip it, but most of us will find some solace in these pages.

The most important principle is that you'll be better off if you can recognize a minor injury before it becomes a serious problem requiring medical attention. The general tendency is for people to assume they can just work through a small strain or minor soreness in a muscle. The quicker you treat the problem with ice, heat, and rest, the sooner you will be back on the roads. Don't take the attitude: "I'll just run through it." In most cases, your body is telling you, in one word: STOP.

A sore muscle is a tired and over-used muscle. It needs some rest. If your legs feel tired and heavy, maybe you should use this day for a quiet walk or swim. Save the run and your legs for another day. When you ignore tired and aching muscles, you will eventually get yourself into injury trouble. Pay attention to your body.

In most cases there will be warning signs leading up to an injury. Pain is a good indication that something is wrong and you better stop and analyze the situation. If it was just a small twinge, maybe a short walk or slower pace with a little light stretching will eliminate the symptom. If the pain continues to bother you, or if it increases, you are probably done for the day at least.

Some light stretching and ice will decrease the chances of a long layoff. When you stretch, avoid stretching the sore muscle. Stretch the ones near it. Slowly ease back into your exercise program while monitoring every little feeling.

A few of the more common injuries are easily discernible. You will recognize black toenails, shin splints, groin pull, basic sore muscles, and sore knees. Others may be more difficult to pinpoint and may actually require a visit to your family doctor or chiropractor.

TOENAILS

Black toenails are probably one of the most common and readily recognized minor injuries. These occur quite often in beginning runners and even though they look awful they're actually not serious—just blocked up blood beneath the nail. Black toenails are usually caused by running shoes that do not fit properly. If your shoes are too tight your toes will bang against the front, especially on any downhill part or your course. You might try trimming your nails closer or wearing a thinner running sock, but in most cases you will need a larger size shoe.

Sometimes a thick sock can get bunched up in the toe area and cause a toenail to bruise. Thick socks may also not let your feet breathe properly. If your socks hold in the moisture and humidity, your toes may swell a little and bruise more easily. Make sure your socks are relatively thin and breathable, and that they fit properly. Long runs on a warm day should also give you warning; hot, sweaty feet are prone to black toenails.

There are home remedies for black toenails, but I would recommend seeing a podiatrist if they are really bothering you.

BLISTERS

Blisters are basically in the same category as black toenails, minor but still aggravating. Abnormal rubbing in your shoe can cause a blister to appear. Sometimes the culprit can be your sock; it is either to thick or could be bunching up in your shoe. Avoid cotton socks because they don't breathe properly and tend to hold the moisture in, leading to blisters and black toenails.

Shoes that don't fit properly can also give you blisters. If your shoe is too big and your foot moves back and forth in the shoe you will work up a blister. Get a shoe that feels snug, but not too tight, and you will more than likely avoid these minor irritations.

SHIN SPLINTS

Although shin splints occur more frequently among novice runners, they can sneak up on seasoned runners a well. Shin splints are aggravating inflammations on either the inside or outside area adjacent to the bone of your lower leg, referred to as the shinbone. They result when the tibias anterior muscle along this bone tears away from its normal position. The calf muscle is generally stronger and tends to overpower the muscle on the front side of the leg, tearing it away. This muscle imbalance will even out as you become more accustomed to running. Changing your running surface, or the camber of the road you run on, can begin the development of shin splints. For instance, you may go on vacation and enjoy a nice run on the beach instead of your normal mileage over city streets. Changing your running course to include a long downhill may also trigger this injury. Even an experienced runner who attacks a new downhill at a faster pace can get in trouble. Switching shoes, or wearing old shoes, can aggravate this injury by changing the position that your heel plants in your stride. Less than 1/4 inch difference can cause shin splints right away.

Fortunately, the cure is quite simple and rest and recovery time is relatively short. Recognizing the injury is pretty easy. The front of your lower leg is sore and if you run your fingers up and down the sides of your shinbone you will feel small tender lumps. What you are feeling are the torn and inflamed muscles.

Icing the area and resting are the best solutions. You might also need new shoes, but be careful not to change your heel position dramatically. Remember not to increase your weekly mileage by more than 10%. This formula should reduce your risk of injury.

HAMSTRINGS

Mere jogging doesn't usually result in a pulled hamstring. This injury is usually associated with sprints. A pulled hamstring is aggravated when you extend your leg straight out. You may be able to continue jogging slowly, keeping your knees bent. Icing the sore area and stretching lightly will get you back in shape quite quickly. Lay off the speed workouts for a while.

ANKLE SPRAIN

The most common cause of a sprain is rolling your ankle over on a step or curb. This abrupt twist puts abnormal tension on the tendons holding your ankle in its proper position—over-stretching or possibly tearing a ligament. You will know the ankle is sprained if you can't put any pressure on your foot. The first thing to do is get an ice pack on the ankle and elevate your foot. If pain persists, you might want to seek medical advice, just to make sure it is not broken. Do not try to run through an ankle injury. You will almost certainly do more damage.

KNEES

Sore knees can usually be fixed pretty easily through a little stretching and rest. A physician, preferably one who is also a runner, should examine anything that feels more serious than "sore."

The knee is very complex; therefore, many things can go wrong with it. Quite a few tendons, ligaments, bones, and cartilage come together in the same area of the knee, including the tibia muscle (lower leg), the femur muscle (thigh), and the patella bone (kneecap). Stretching the calf muscle and treating it with ice should clear up minor soreness. Stretching the calf muscle will take some of the tension off the tendons that attach to heel and knee, simultaneously reducing soreness. If soreness persists or worsens, try changing your shoes and running on a level surface before heading to the sports injury clinic.

ILIOTIBIAL

Pain along the outside area of your knee and hip is usually associated with an inflammation of the Iliotibial band tendon. Many times this can be caused by running on a cambered road, which puts stress on one side of your body by encouraging it to compensate for an uneven surface. Running laps on a track can sometimes cause problems with the Iliotibial tendon. One leg being slightly shorter than the other can also strain it. Putting a prescribed heel lift in one shoe can correct a body structure problem—and running on even surfaces will certainly help.

GROIN

Injuries in the groin area can be aggravating because they sometimes last a long time. The adductor muscles, located in your inner thigh, are the ones that get pulled. Pulls can sometimes result from running on slippery or icy streets (which I told you not to do) because as you plant your food it tends to slip backwards. The adductor tries to stop this slippage and you end up with a groin pull. Again check your shoes for wear and proper fit.

The slightest twinge in the groin should be a signal to rest. Don't even think of trying to run through a groin pull; it just won't work. Light stretching and ice are the best cure—along with some time off.

ACHILLES TENDON

Achilles tendonitis, if recognized early, can usually be corrected with an easy stretch of your calf muscle. As I mentioned earlier, your Achilles tendon attaches your heel to your calf muscle. When the calf gets tight or overly contracted it will put pressure on the Achilles tendon by pulling on it. Tight hamstrings will cause the same problem. The best remedy is to stretch the calf and hamstrings gently. If the pain doesn't clear up after a little rest, rest some more and stretch lightly. Check your shoes for too much cushioning or too low a heel and too stiff a forefoot.

Reduce your running and cut out uphill work, which puts an extra strain on your Achilles tendon. You don't want to mess with an Achilles tendon. If yours pops, you will know it and your down time will be considerable.

PLANTAR FASCIITIS

Plantar fasciitis is a tearing of the plantar fascia, which connect the toes to the heel. It is usually felt just in front of the heel before the arch. If the tear is at the heel bone, you could develop heel spurs, which are visible on an x-ray. When you wake in the morning and take your first couple of steps toward the bathroom, you will feel soreness in your foot. After walking and a little massage, it will tend to not bother you as much, but you still should lay off the running until it heals. Excessive pronation or shoes with too much bend in the arch area could be the culprits. Talk to your running shoe store specialist.

ICE

Many runners get confused about the proper use of ice and heat in treating an injury. Ice brings down the inflammation by restricting the flow of blood and heat increases the circulation, which carries away waste products.

The question is when to apply each. Right after an injury, apply ice for 20 minutes and repeat several times. On the following day, apply heat for 20 minutes at a stretch, repeating several times. Two days after the injury, you can alternate between ice and heat, which will continue to reduce the inflammation and flush out the injured area.

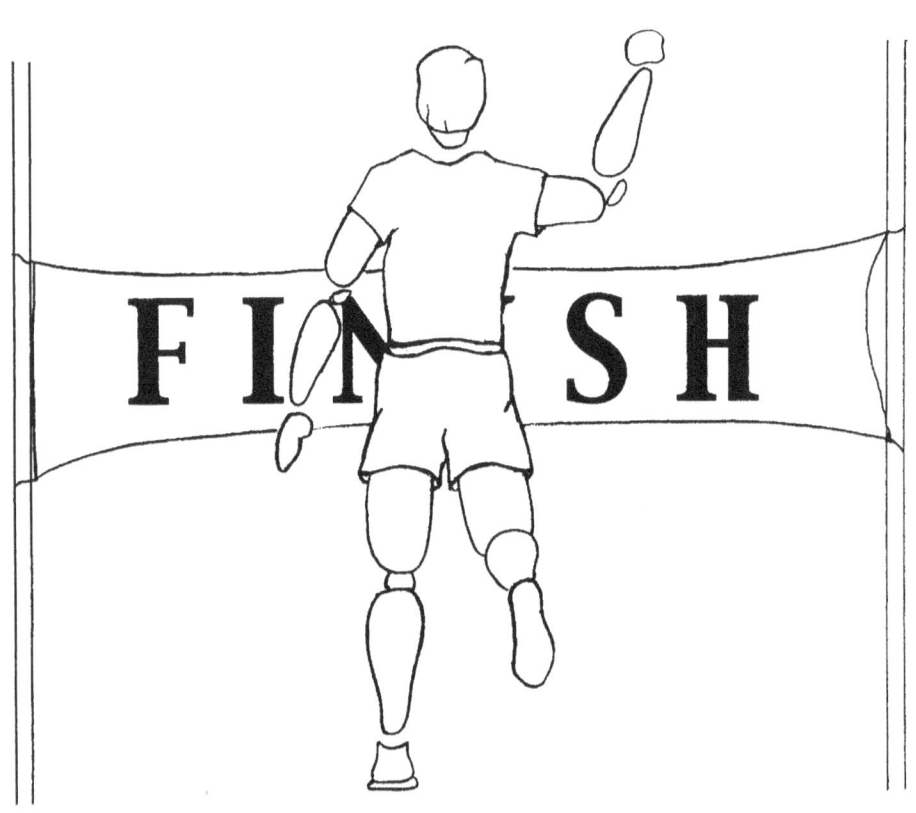

Competition

You may begin thinking about competition during your training regimen. Competing is not for everyone, but in running, the term can take on widely variant meanings—depending on the level of interest and personality of the runner. For some, winning is the ultimate goal; for others just attempting to finish is enough. The beauty of running is that there are many degrees of competition between these two extremes—upfront runner and last finisher. Personally I prefer to compete in my own age group. The rest of the race can fly by—and it usually does—but position in my group of runners is what's important to me.

After months of working hard at getting yourself in shape, you may want to seek an objective measure of what you have accomplished. You feel and look great, but you may want to test yourself against your peers. A weekend 5K or 10K is the perfect way to see where you will finish against a bunch of other runners. Where you are in your training will determine which type or length of race you'll want to enter. For beginners, a 5K is the perfect place to start. *5K* stands for 5 kilometers or 5000 meters or 3.1 miles. A *10K* is double that length—10 kilometers, 10,000 meters, or 6.2 miles.

Pick a local race with a nice, easy course—preferably over a scenic and enjoyable route. Don't change your diet the week before a race, but continue to eat the healthy foods you've learned about in this book. I've known people who bulk up on fruit trying to carbo-load the week before and end up in line for the port-a-potty. Stick with a light snack, like a piece of toast and one cup of coffee, and save your real meal for post race. Concentrate on the carbohydrates that you have been eating—the good ones.

Grab a friend or someone you have been training with and decide which race to enter. Try to pre-register so you can avoid some of the last-minute rush and confusion at sign-in. You will still have to go to a designated area to pick up your race packet and t-shirt, if you ordered one. In this packet will be your race number and a few other items that vary from race to race. Make sure everything is correct on your race number, for example, name, age group, and gender. Arriving early will allow you a short warm-up and time to get in a little stretching. Most important—locate the port-a-potties because the line will grow the closer it gets to race time. Try to get all of that out of way early. Take your sweats, and any other items you won't be needing during the race, to your car and head for the starting area.

Lining up at the start line is important and, unfortunately, not enough people pay attention to where they are in the group. The runners in the very front will be the eventual leaders and will be running under 5 minutes per mile. You definitely don't want to get in their way. The next group will be the 5–6 minute-per-mile runners and you will probably want to avoid them also. Move yourself back around the 8–10 per mile folks and you will have a good start. You can usually recognize this group because they are all talking and laughing and not really taking the race too seriously. This is right where you want to be. Now take a few minutes to check your shoelaces, double knot them, take a few deep breaths, and get relaxed. The gun is about to go off.

On race day everybody is excited and a little more pumped up than usual. This will carry over to the race start. Don't try to go out with everybody else; run your own race. You know what your pace is, so plan to stick with it. If you don't, you'll find yourself burning out way before you want to. Once the race starts, move along with everybody until you attain your specific pace. Concentrate on not getting pulled along by the surge of the crowd.

A timekeeper will usually announce the split times at the first mile. If you don't see one, watch for a mile marker and check your time. You can adjust up or down to maintain your pace. If you had a good start, without too much pushing and jostling, I'll bet you'll be ahead of your forecast at the first mile. That's all right, just slow it down for the next 2.1 miles and you will be fine.

Settle in now and look around, take notice of your company. How are they doing? How old are they? Male or female? Pick out somebody who appears to be running similar to you and follow that person for a while. Maybe you will feel strong enough to gradually slip by him or her without overexerting. Approaching the finish line, make sure you finish in the correct shoot; it is usually apparent. No need to try and pass someone in the shoot. It looks bad and the race is supposed to be run on the course. Get your time and head for the water and other refreshments. You have earned them.

The awards can't be given out until everyone finishes and even then it takes time to tabulate the different category awards. Relax and do some light stretching while you have a moment. Once they finally tally up all the times they will usually award the overall winners (1st through 3rd) for both male and female. Next they will go down all the age-group division winners (1st through 5th). These are usually broken down into five-year spans (25–29, 30–34, etc.). Get your ribbon and celebrate.

Old! Why are we referred to as old? Why can't we just gain in years? In Spanish the literal translation of *"Cuantos años tiene usted?"* is "How many years do you have?" Much better. We are only as old as we feel. Fortunately, we can feel better through exercise and therefore feel and act younger. So do you want to change your life and feel better? Eliminate the word *old* from your vocabulary and add some words like *ageless, healthy, stamina,* and *youthful.* Running is one of the few sports in which you can look forward to entering each new age group as the youngster.

No matter what you call it, aging is still difficult. For years I couldn't accept the fact that I was actually becoming slower. I would lie to myself. My old run of five miles that would normally take 35 minutes was now taking 40 minutes, but I was still running 35 and calling it five miles. It's hard to adjust, but the sooner you can accept that fact of life, the sooner you can begin training anew. Running—so it has been said—helps you age more slowly.

Now that I have accepted my changing position in the walk of life, my running has taken a definite turn for the better. My training and racing times have improved. I'm not quite to the seven-minute benchmark I used to click off, but I'm achieving times that allow me to feel optimistic about my training and results. It must be pretty funny to watch a 60-year-old runner doing speed work on the track.

This improvement in my running shows up in my racing; but more important, it creates a better outlook on life itself, improving the way I approach each new day. This is the attitude you want to develop—a positive feeling about yourself and your future. When you see changes taking place, you have to feel good about what you have accomplished. You look better, your clothes fit better, you eat better—all of which directly affect your health and well-being. You don't have to win the race to experience all these emotions. Just being there should make you feel great about yourself.

Of course, these positive attitudes will carry over into your home life and your work place. It's one thing for me to be telling you about mental and physical changes, but when you actually experience them you will be very proud of your accomplishments. So let's get out there and "burn" some more calories to get in shape for the next race.

Great Runs

For many years I was associated with *Runner's World Magazine*. I wrote a couple of books that mapped out and described where to run in over 200 cities throughout the United States. The first books were titled *The Great American Runner's Guides.* One covered the western states and the other the east coast. *Runner's World* marketed and distributed these books for several years, while I proceeded to work on the mid-west and southern cities. Unfortunately, before I finished the project, *Runner's World* and I parted ways; still, the experience was very rewarding.

The books were designed to aid traveling runners while they were away from home. Running in a large, strange city can be very intimidating—not to mention scary. Finding a safe location, close to your hotel, where you can get in a few miles is trying and difficult in some cities. Most hotel employees are not runners, and even if they are, they run in their own neighborhoods and know nothing about running downtown. So I tried to visit every average sized city in the U.S. and map out a 10-mile run from the local hotels. Back in those days, everyone ran 10 miles a day, seven days a week. These runs can be shortened to fit the individual runner, but 10 miles is the standard.

In this chapter, I have re-introduced a few of my favorite runs from *The Great American Runner's Guide*—eastern and western editions. The hotels have been excluded because most have changed ownership, name, logo, and sometimes reputation.

Running on city streets should be avoided if possible. In most cities there will be much better choices to be found along rivers, ocean beaches, through the woods and on many college and university campuses.

A couple things will happen to you after you have read by book and followed my thoughts and instructions toward altering your lifestyle. First and foremost, of course, you will become an athlete and actually enjoy exercise. Second you will be able to run on vacations or while traveling with your business.

To me, there is nothing that compares to running in a strange city and introducing myself to new paths and trails that crisscross all the new horizons across our country.

Obviously, I can't include all the great runs that I have experienced but hopefully, these will get you started in the right direction. Now that you are fit and healthy, I hope that you will discover many new trails in your life.

Let Private Sudz be your guide.

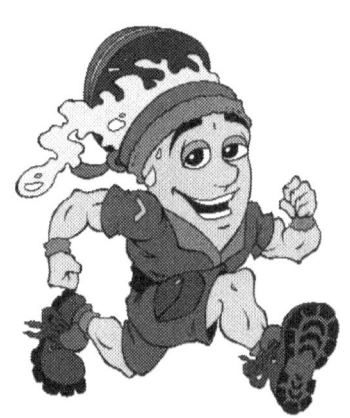

BAR HARBOR, MAINE

Plan to stay awhile. There are over fifty miles of carefully groomed carriage roads and one hundred and twenty miles of hiking trails in Acadia National Park on Mount Desert Island. The trails in this park are the nicest I have run on anywhere. I definitely have to return for more of the best running I've ever enjoyed.

Make sure you get out to Eagle Lake—approximately three miles to the lake and about four miles around. It is absolutely beautiful and crystal clear.

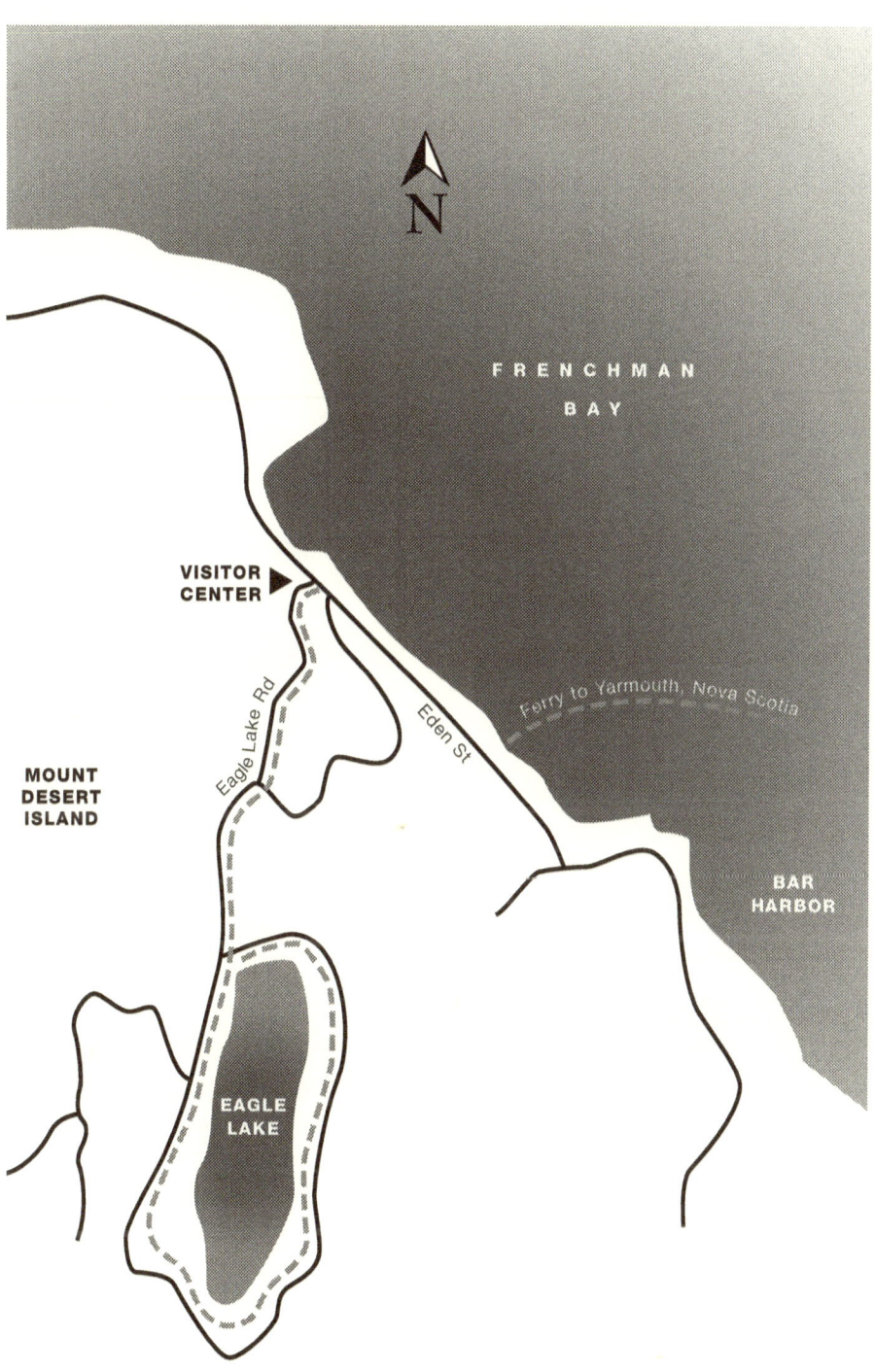

FRENCHMAN
BAY

VISITOR
CENTER

Ferry to Yarmouth, Nova Scotia

Eagle Lake Rd

Eden St

MOUNT
DESERT
ISLAND

BAR
HARBOR

EAGLE
LAKE

PHILADELPHIA, PENNSYLVANIA

Fairmont Park borders the Schuylkill River on both sides for as many miles as you can possibly complete in one day of running. Starting at the Philadelphia Museum of Art you will be impressed right away by the majestic old structures on your left that make up Boat House Row.

I returned from my run about 12:15 p.m. and it seemed like the entire city was vacating in their various running shoes and gear. I might mention it was the day after a snow storm and the temperature was about twenty degrees Fahrenheit with ice and snow on the trail, but it didn't seem to hinder or slow the running masses.

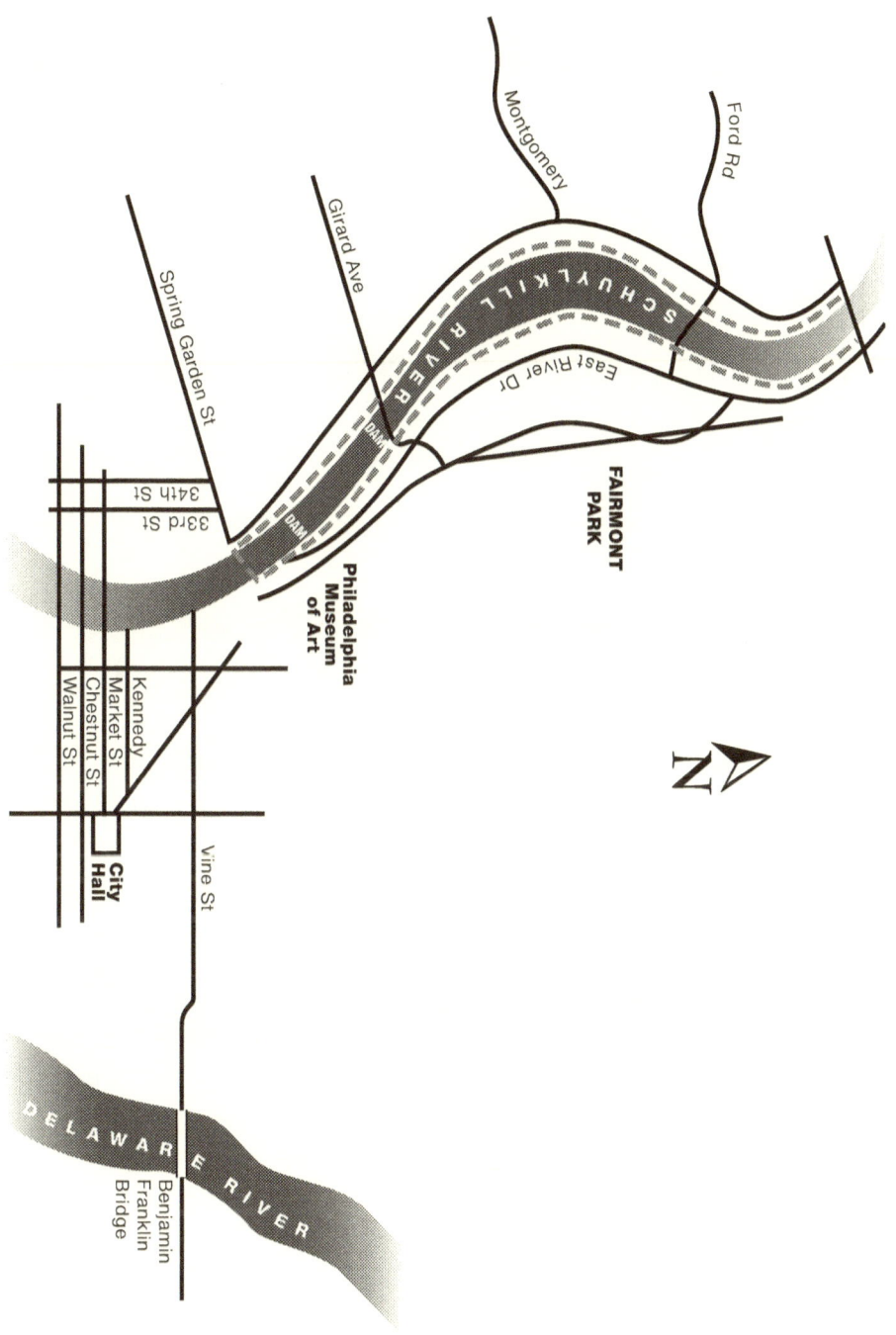

Montgomery

Ford Rd

Girard Ave

Spring Garden St

SCHUYLKILL RIVER

East River Dr

FAIRMONT
PARK

34th St

33rd St

DAM

DAM

Philadelphia
Museum
of Art

Kennedy

Market St

Chestnut St

Walnut St

City
Hall

Vine St

N

DELAWARE RIVER

Benjamin
Franklin
Bridge

BOSTON, MASSACHUSSETS

Boston is a serious runner's city. With the great tradition of the Boston Marathon, Bostonians can hardly avoid at least *thinking* about running. The Charles River is the place to begin. A paved trail lines both sides of the river and, depending on which bridge you cross, you can run a four-, seven-, or ten-mile loop.

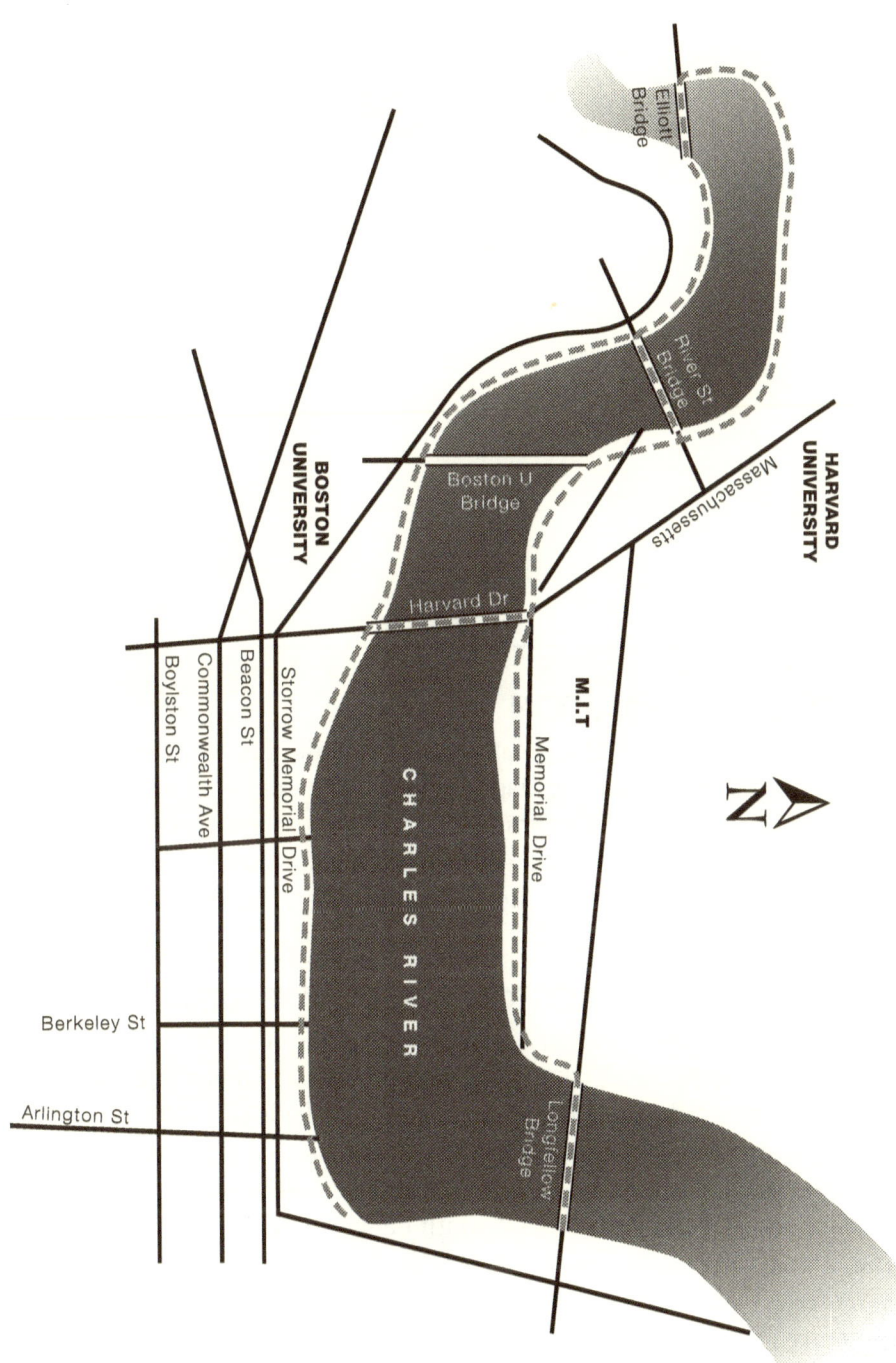

SEATTLE, WASHINGTON

Downtown Seattle has a great place to run right along Elliott Bay. An early morning run out to the Happy Hooker is the perfect way to start the day. This Happy Hooker is a fishing and bait shop at the north end of your run and a perfect place to make your turn around. Now head back to Pike's Place Market at the south end, stop for some coffee, and enjoy all the activity in the market place.

UNIVERSITY OF WASHINGTON /GREEN LAKE AREA

Out of downtown Seattle, take Aurora Avenue north into Green Lake Park. You'll find plenty of parking around the lake and a public track in the southeast corner. Running distance around the lake is close to three miles.

If you get tired of Green Lake, you can run east on Ravenna Boulevard for about a mile to Ravenna Park for some great trail running.

Leaving the park and running south on Seventeenth Avenue for a mile and a half will take you to the University of Washington campus. Seventeenth is a great run by itself—lots of trees and fraternity and sorority houses. The Burke-Gilman Trail runs through the campus. You can follow it northeast for as long as you can run.

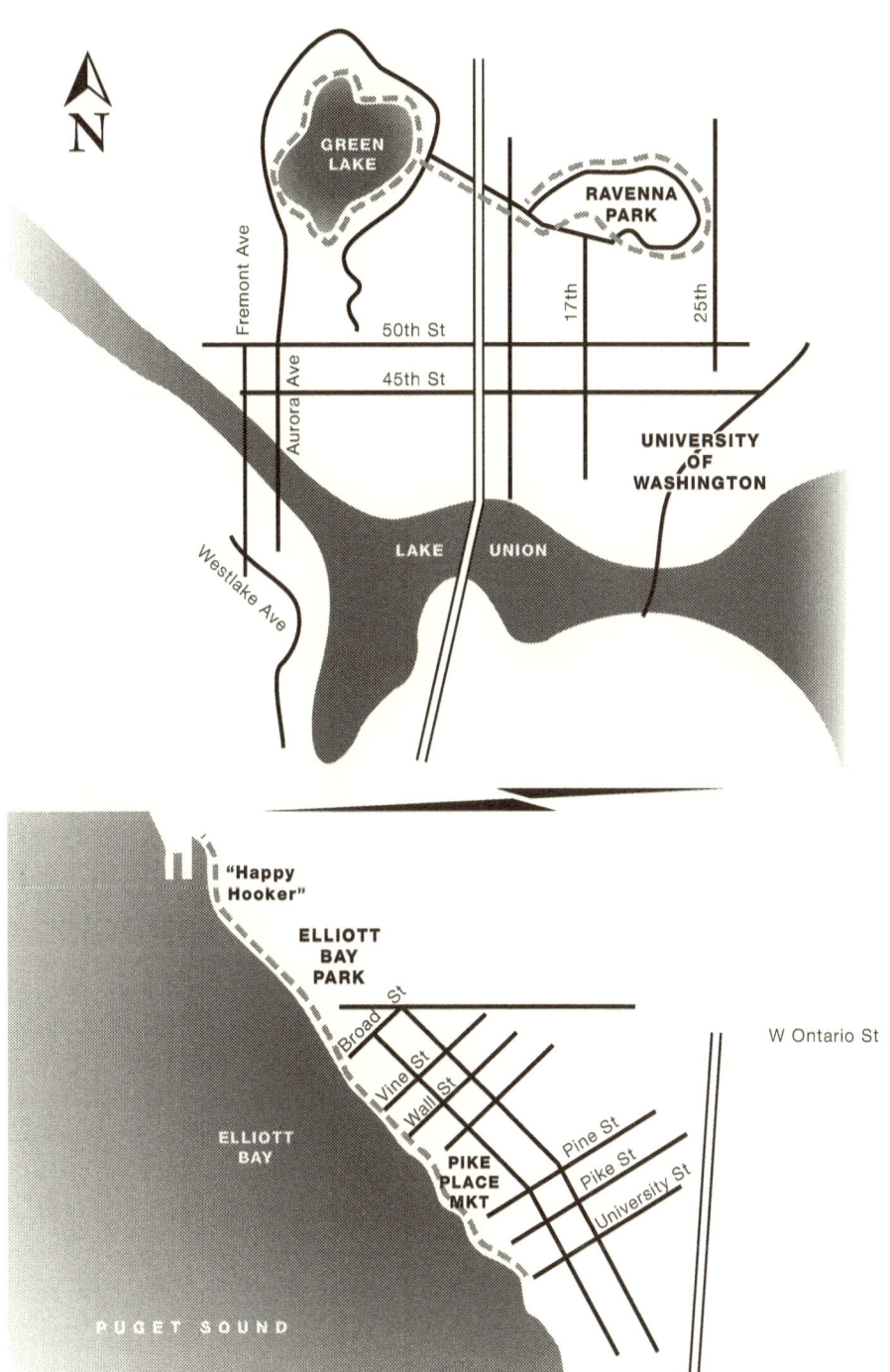

N

GREEN
LAKE

RAVENNA
PARK

Fremont Ave

17th

25th

50th St

Aurora Ave

45th St

UNIVERSITY
OF
WASHINGTON

Westlake Ave

LAKE   UNION

"Happy
Hooker"

ELLIOTT
BAY
PARK

Broad St

W Ontario St

Vine St

Wall St

ELLIOTT
BAY

Pine St

Pike St

PIKE
PLACE
MKT

University St

PUGET SOUND

Great Runs

DENVER, COLORADO

Surprisingly, downtown Denver has its own special place to run, away from the traffic of the city. Cherry Creek runs south to the Denver Country Club and you can bypass the golf course to get more mileage. Running north on the creek trail will take you to Confluence Park where the South Platte River joins Cherry Creek. You can run north or south. Plan to end your run at Confluence Park where you can enjoy a Starbucks while watching all the activity on the river. There, you can usually find a few adventurous souls practicing their capsizing rolls in the falls, which should get your attention.

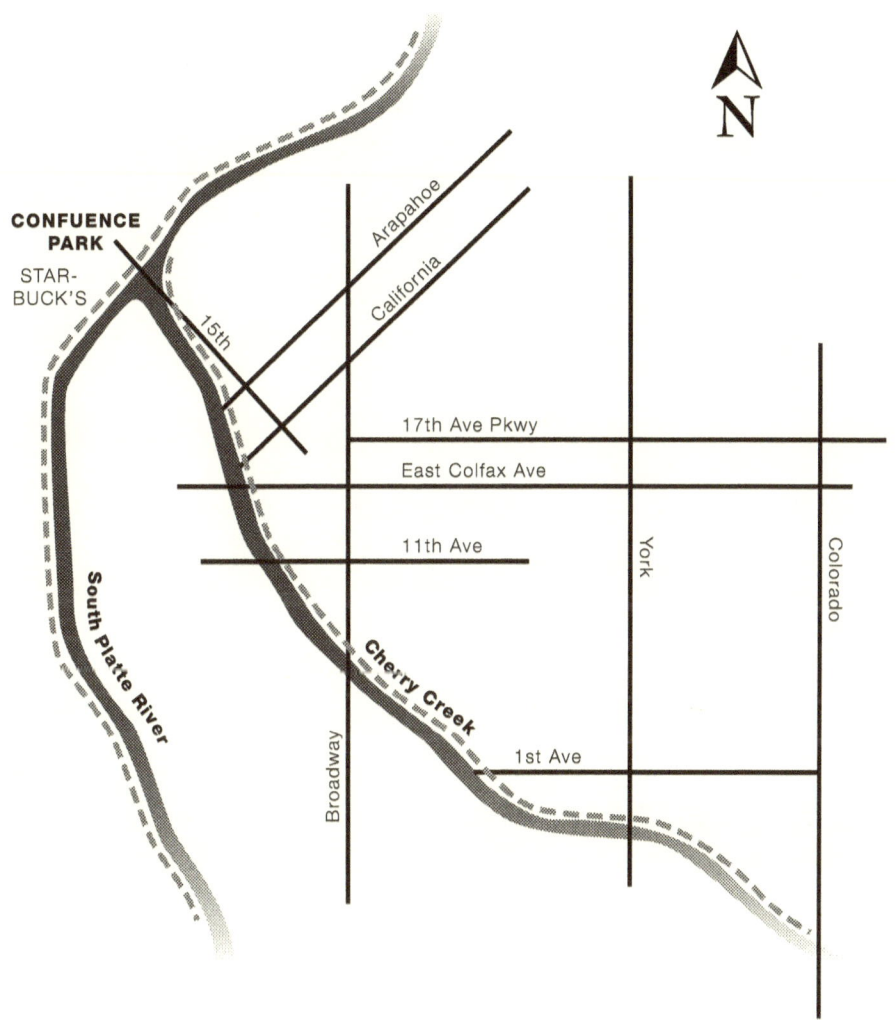

N

CONFUENCE
PARK
STAR-
BUCK'S

Arapahoe

California

15th

17th Ave Pkwy

East Colfax Ave

11th Ave

South Platte River

Cherry Creek

Broadway

York

Colorado

1st Ave

EUGENE, OREGON

While in this city you may get the feeling that the river was formed and the buildings and streets were all constructed with running in mind. The trail along the Willamette River is certainly one of the most beautiful runs I've enjoyed anywhere. There are many loops, bridges, and "Pre's Trail," named in honor of Steve Prefontaine, all through Alton Baker Park.

South of town another great running area is called Amazon Park, including a one-mile rolling track where you can check your times.

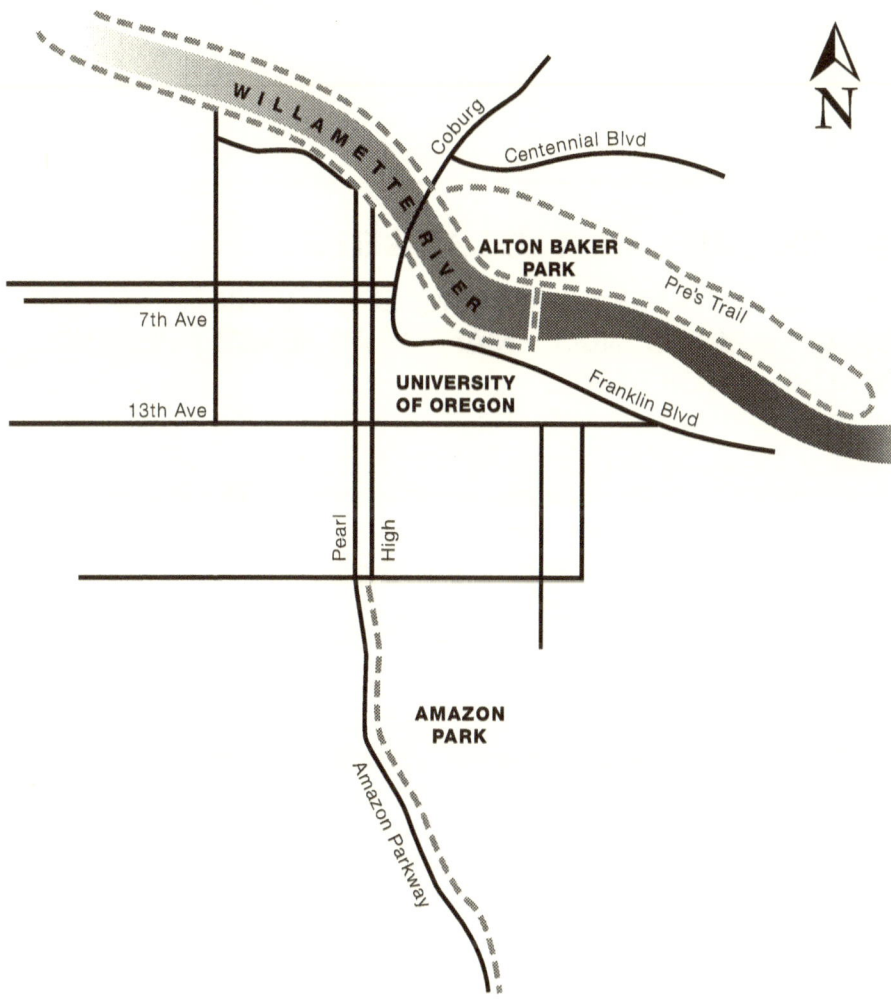

BEACH CITIES, WEST LOS ANGELES

PACIFIC PALISADES • SANTA MONICA • VENICE • MARINA DEL REY • EL SEGUNDO • MANHATTAN BEACH • REDONDO BEACH • PALOS VERDES

Starting at Sunset Boulevard on the Pacific Coast Highway you can run south all the way to Palos Verdes. Unfortunately, Malibu and Topanga Beach don't have a bike trail for running, but the southern trek will keep you satisfied. Save your surfing for another day.

Once you reach State Beach on your run south, you may want to venture up to the Palisades Bluff and run along Ocean Avenue. Another great run is along San Vicente Boulevard to the east. Coming back down San Vicente you may want to try out the steps at Adelaide. It has become the "in" spot for stair walking and running. I last counted one hundred and eighty-six steps, although the number seems to change every time I run them.

Continuing along the bike trail on the coast through Santa Monica and Venice you will eventually reach Washington Boulevard where you will have to run east a few blocks and enter Marina Del Rey. After a nice, enjoyable run past all the magnificent boat and yachts you will head south again. El Segundo, Manhattan and Redondo offer great running all year long, but the scenery is much better during the summer months.

Maps of these Beach Cities runs continuee on pages 102 and 103.

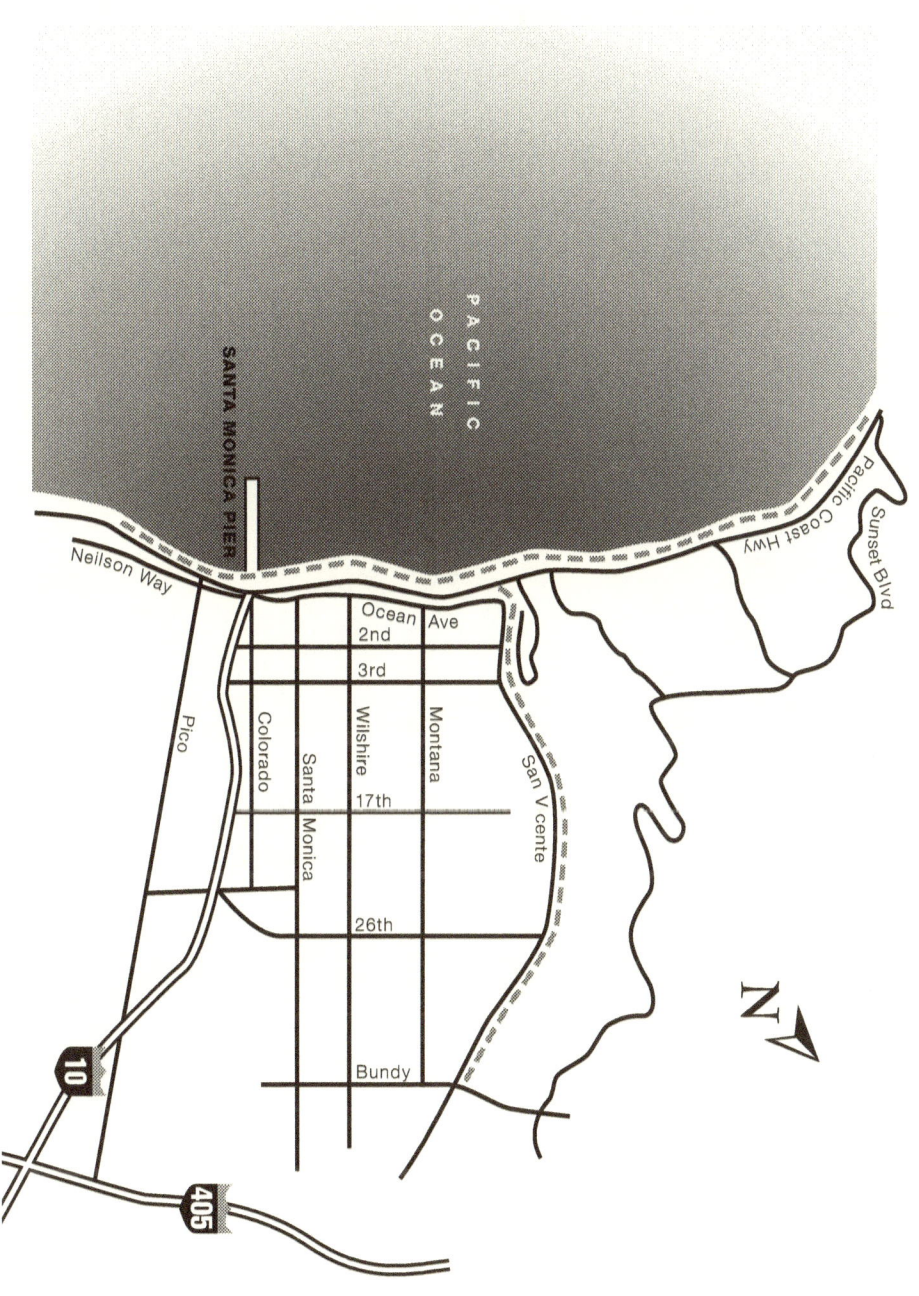

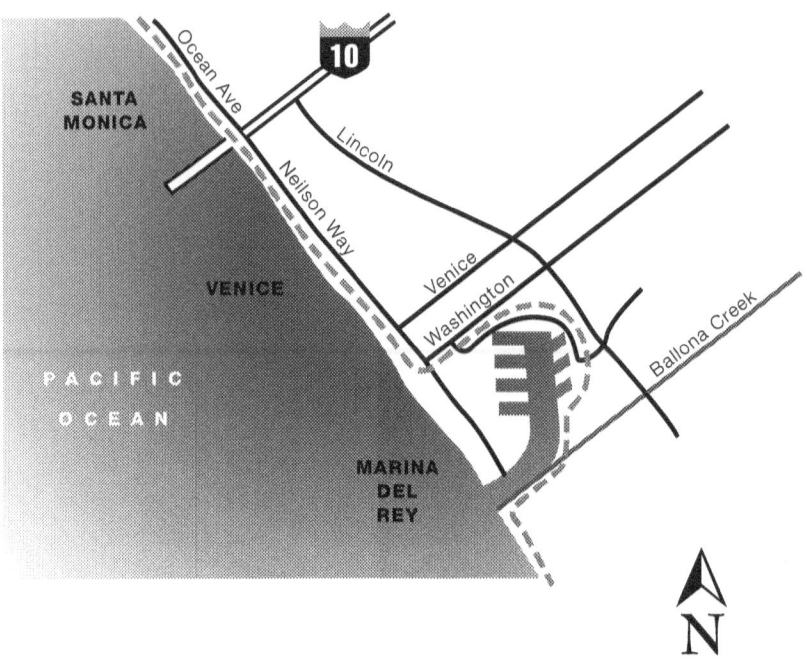

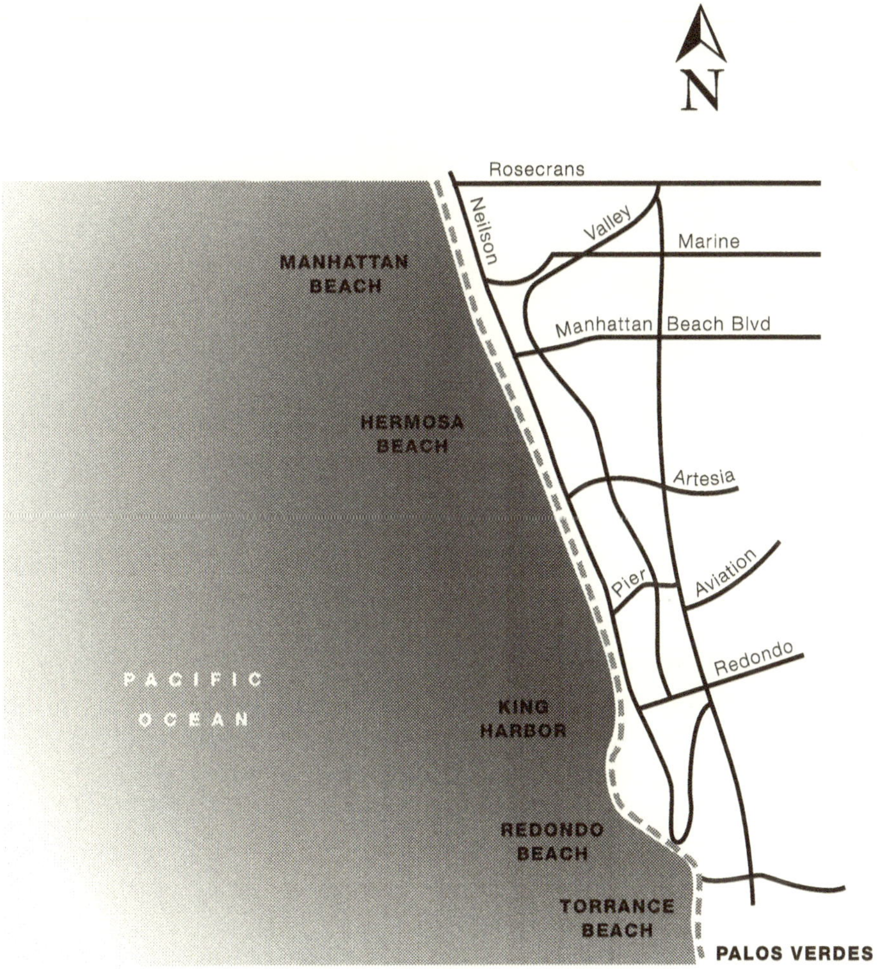

Rosecrans

Neilson

Valley

Marine

**MANHATTAN
BEACH**

Manhattan Beach Blvd

**HERMOSA
BEACH**

Artesia

Pier

Aviation

**PACIFIC
OCEAN**

Redondo

**KING
HARBOR**

**REDONDO
BEACH**

**TORRANCE
BEACH**

PALOS VERDES

ANCHORAGE, ALASKA

Try this great run close to downtown Anchorage. Follow a couple twists and turns and then take Bootlegger Cove right to Westchester Lagoon. From the lagoon you can continue along Cook Inlet all the way to the airport. This trail is fantastic, but not to be outdone by the trail heading east. Running east gives you an opportunity to cruise through three campuses on your journey: Anchorage Community College, University of Alaska, and Alaska Pacific University.

The scenery on both runs is spectacular so you will have to stay an extra day to get in all the necessary shoe time.

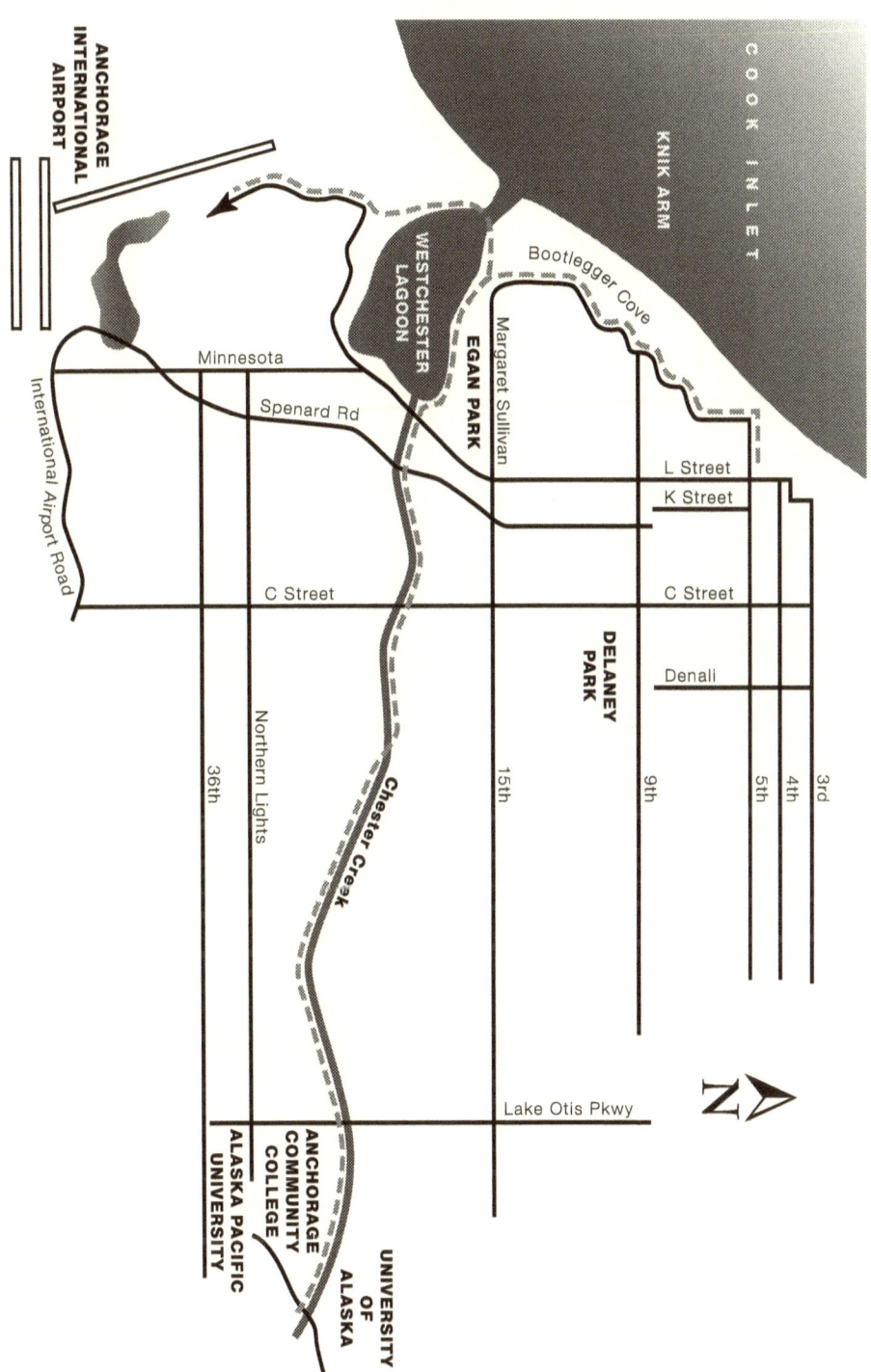

ANCHORAGE
INTERNATIONAL
AIRPORT

COOK INLET

KNIK ARM

WESTCHESTER
LAGOON

Bootlegger Cove

EGAN PARK

Margaret Sullivan

Minnesota

International Airport Road

Spenard Rd

L Street

K Street

C Street

C Street

DELANEY
PARK

Denali

36th

Northern Lights

Chester Creek

15th

9th

5th

4th

3rd

Lake Otis Pkwy

N

ALASKA PACIFIC
UNIVERSITY

ANCHORAGE
COMMUNITY
COLLEGE

UNIVERSITY
OF
ALASKA

HONOLULU, HAWAII

This is it! The place where every runner's dream comes true. The temperatures in the morning and evening are pleasant, a little warm during the middle of the day. A cooling trade wind usually blows. You can't beat running through Kahala, surrounded by foliage and the slight fragrance of plumeria trees penetrating your awakened senses.

Starting at Kapiolani Park, which is a fantastic run all by itself, you can reach Kahala by two different paths. Turning left on Monserrat Avenue will take you away from the ocean and around Diamond Head the back way. I prefer to run straight ahead on Diamond Head Road. This will take you up a slight hill and down the other side to Black Point. Continue straight ahead on Kahala Avenue all the way to the Waialae Golf Course. This is a seven- or eight-mile run you will never forget.

Back in Waikiki you can enjoy a nice run along the Ala Wai canal. It's fun to watch the outrigger canoe paddling clubs training in the canal.

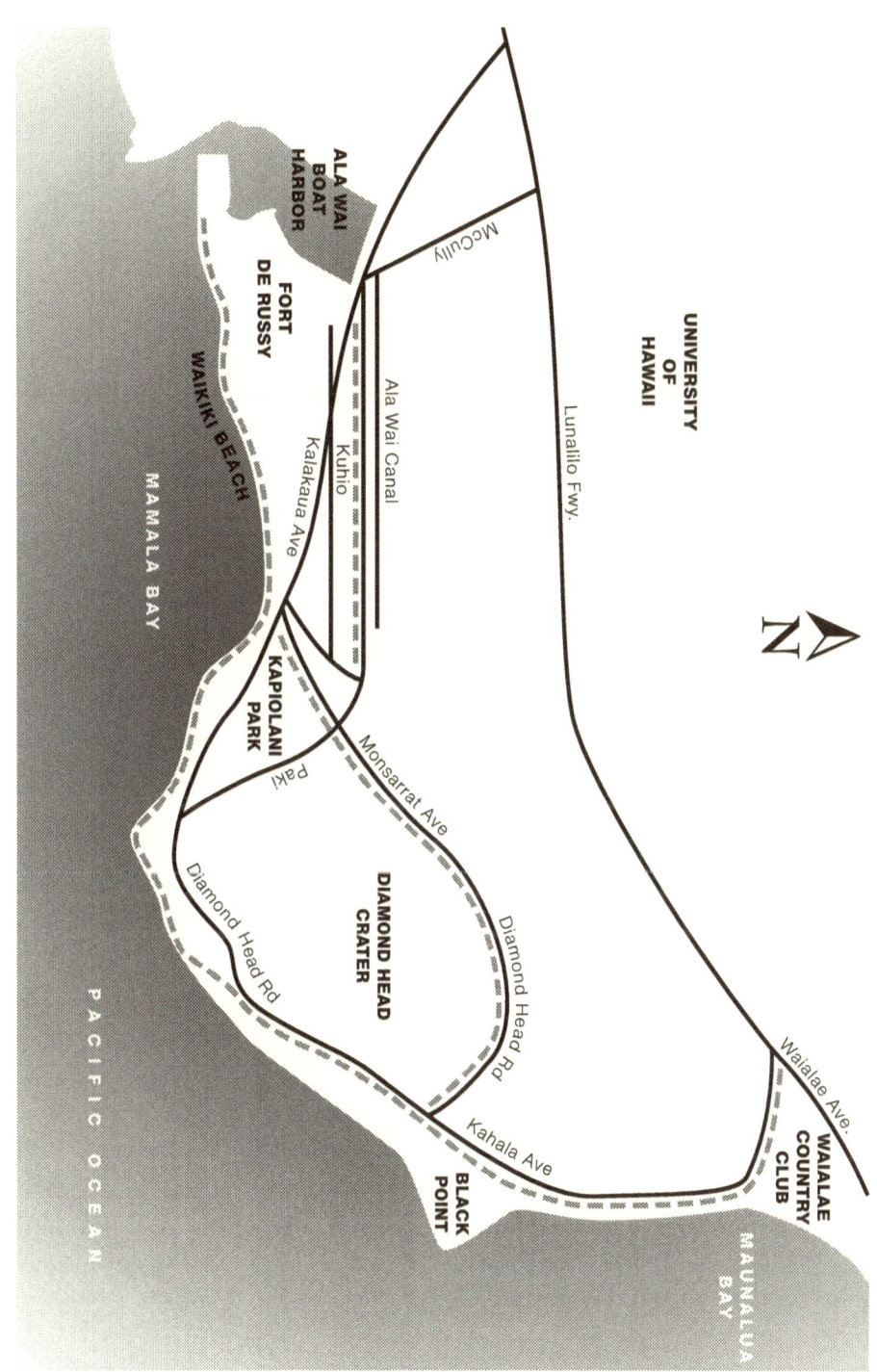

ALA WAI
BOAT
HARBOR

FORT
DE RUSSY

WAIKIKI BEACH

MAMALA BAY

McCully

Ala Wai Canal

Kalakaua Ave

Kuhio

UNIVERSITY
OF
HAWAII

Lunalilo Fwy.

N

KAPIOLANI
PARK

Paki

Monsarrat Ave

DIAMOND HEAD
CRATER

Diamond Head Rd

Diamond Head Rd

Waialae Ave.

WAIALAE
COUNTRY
CLUB

PACIFIC OCEAN

Kahala Ave

BLACK
POINT

MAUNALUA
BAY

SAN DIEGO, CALIFORNIA

San Diego Bay is wonderful for running. North Harbor Drive will take you from Shelter Island to Harbor Island and then a little farther south. You'll end up along the Embarcadero, which has lots of shops and restaurants for your after-run pleasure.

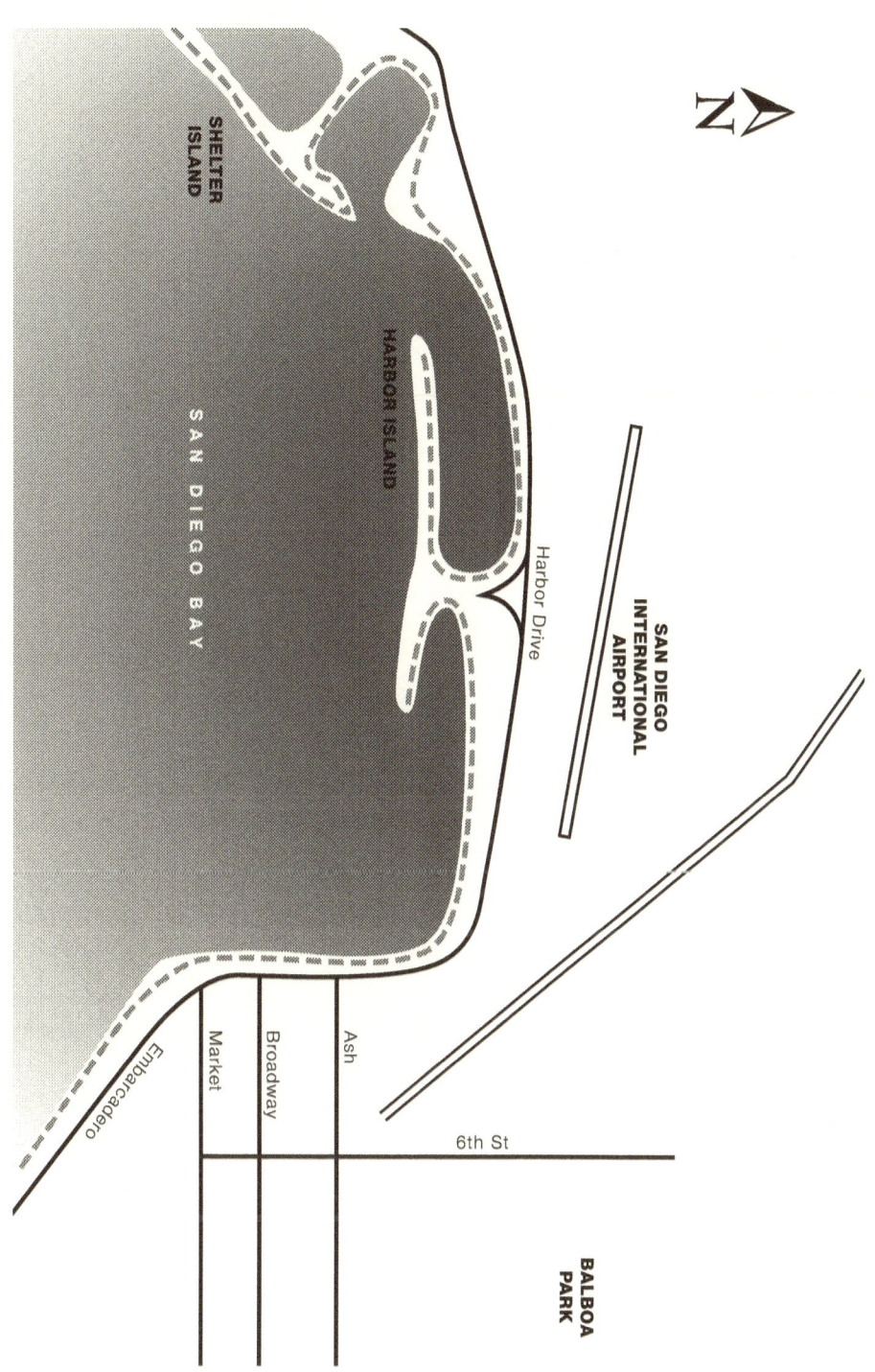

N

SHELTER
ISLAND

HARBOR ISLAND

SAN DIEGO BAY

Harbor Drive

SAN DIEGO
INTERNATIONAL
AIRPORT

Embarcadero

Market

Broadway

Ash

6th St

BALBOA
PARK

SAN FRANCISCO, CALIFORNIA

I've experienced three great runs in the San Francisco area, though I'm sure there are many more.

Running along the Embarcadero in the city itself is a great way to enjoy the San Francisco Bay. Starting at the south end, you can work your way around and end up heading west toward the Golden Gate Bridge. This run can be crowded on pleasant summer days, but still well worth the effort.

The other two runs (not on this map) are located near the San Francisco Airport. As a matter of fact, the first one starts right next to the runway. You can follow a trail south to Coyote Point and then a little further to one of South Bay's yacht harbors.

In the foothills above the airport you'll be surprised to find an excellent run along Sawyer Camp Trail. The trail follows the water from Crystal Springs Reservoir to the northwest end of San Andreas Lake.

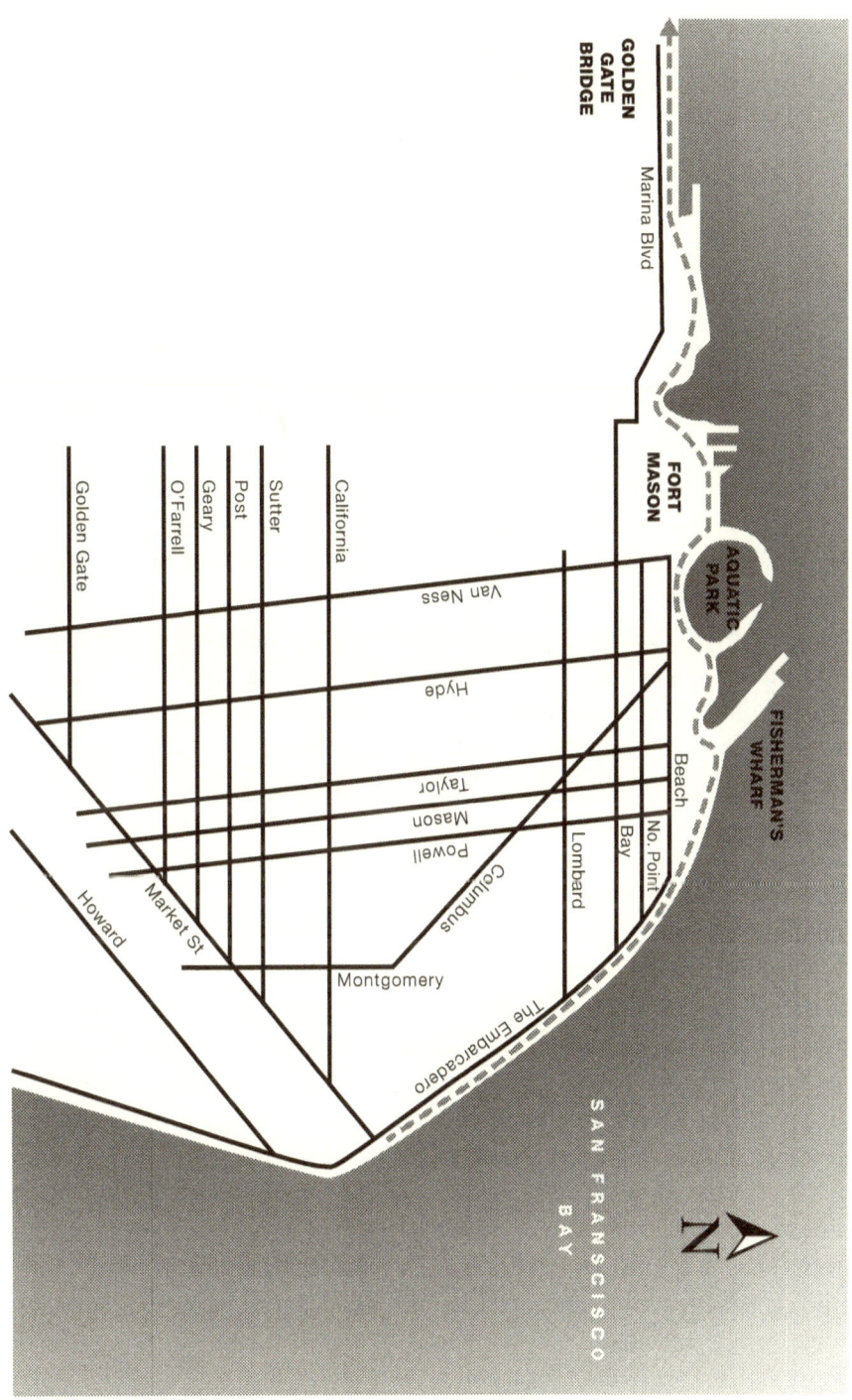

JOCKEY HOLLOW AND MORRISTOWN, NEW JERSEY

If you neither walk or run, this is the perfect place to begin. The Morristown and Madison area offers trails way beyond your expectations. This area is one of the few places in which I have seen road signs alerting the drivers to joggers on the road. The sign says, "Bicycles and joggers in roadway," but it should say "Please joggers stay off road." These country roads are the loveliest I have seen anywhere, but they are too narrow for two cars and one jogger. Enjoy the scenery from your car and read on to discover where to jog free from noise, cars, and exhaust fumes. You will only have to watch for deer, rabbits, squirrels, and probably a few other enlightened runners.

Jockey Hollow: Talk about taking a journey through history. This run will certainly take you there. Jockey Hollow is the historical site of George Washington's long winter stay during the Revolutionary War. I don't suggest making this run is a red sweatshirt, as I did. It gives you the eerie feeling that some Continental soldiers might be gunning for the last of the "red coats." Plenty of parking at the visitor center and you can follow the paved road around for a great run. In summer, I prefer to follow the footpaths through the trees. There are posted trail guides about every half mile, which makes it easy for you to choose your route as you weave around and up and down what may well become one of your favorite runs.

On the other side of the valley a different park deserves your attention now that you are warmed up to trail running. Loantaka Park is accessible from Blue Mill Road and there is a nice parking area from which you can enjoy this run on both sides of Blue Mill Road. Lots of deer will be watching you.

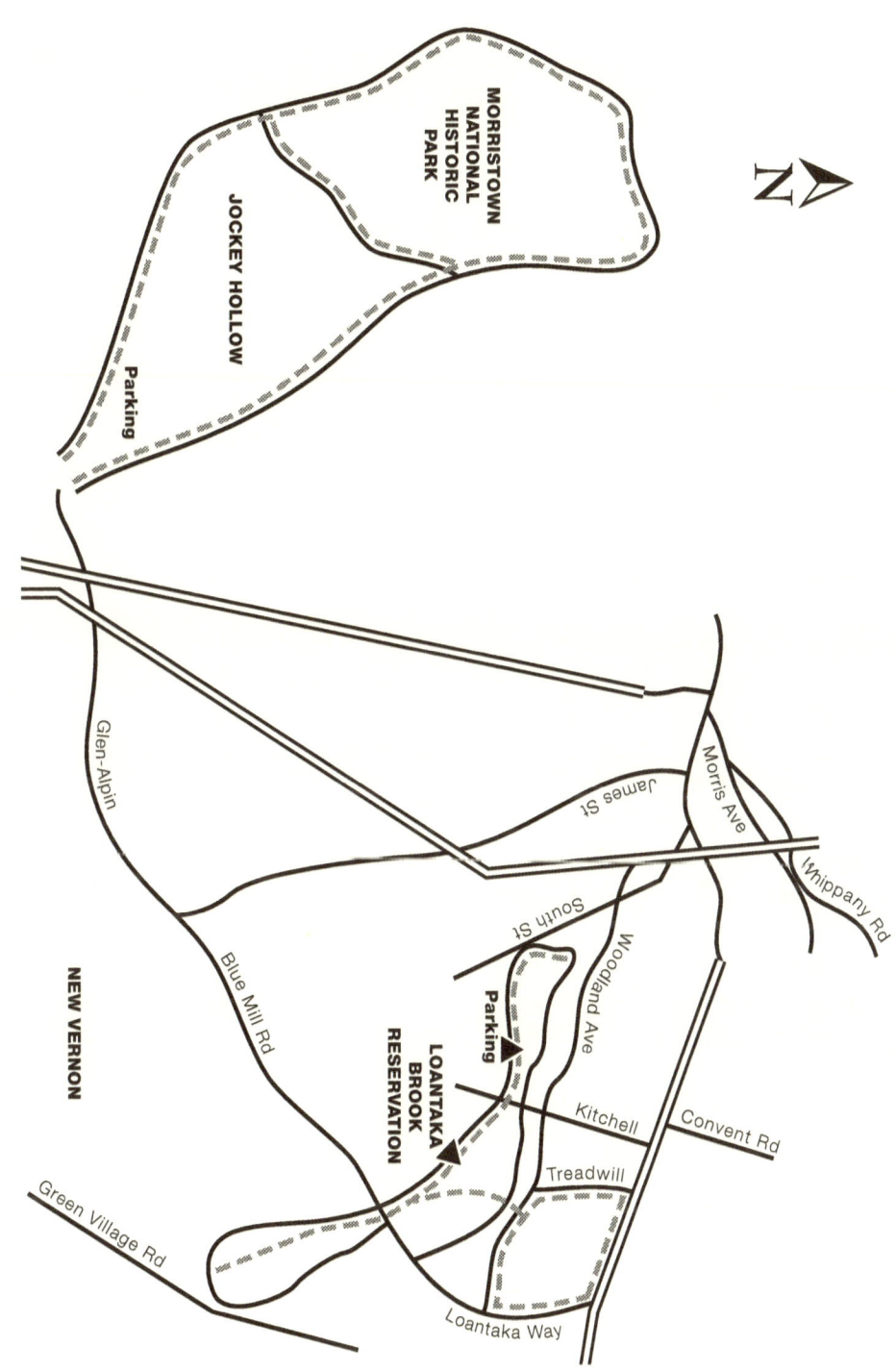

MORRISTOWN NATIONAL HISTORIC PARK

JOCKEY HOLLOW

Parking

N

Glen-Alpin

James St

Morris Ave

Whippany Rd

South St

Blue Mill Rd

NEW VERNON

Parking

Woodland Ave

LOANTAKA BROOK RESERVATION

Kitchell

Convent Rd

Treadwill

Green Village Rd

Loantaka Way

Great Runs

CENTRAL PARK IN NEW YORK, NEW YORK

You probably wouldn't think that New York City could be one of your favorite places to run, but Central Park is thoroughly enjoyable. You might come gliding out of the park singing "I love New York," or barking at a hot dog vender, "Gimme a dawg, buster" with a smile on your face.

Central Park stretches north from 59th Street all the way to 110th in Harlem. It also lies between Fifth Avenue and Eight Avenue. Getting to the park, pedestrian traffic will be heavy and moving fast. The walking pace of New Yorkers will allow you an excellent warm-up for your run.

A good location to start is at the corner of 59th and Fifth Avenue. The park itself has plenty of trails for a run of any distance, but I prefer the total loop on the main road, which is six miles. If you want to avoid the "Great Hill," you can cut off around 102nd on the east side and wind down to about 90th on the west side. If you are alone or approaching evening, it is probably a good idea to take the cut-off to avoid any problems.

The reservoir is a very popular area. One and a half miles circles the lake. You will find it fairly well lighted and patrolled. Of course, on the weekends, this area will be crowded, but moving along at a good pace. Out in the park will be baseball, frisbees, skaters, dog walkers, bikes, and just about anything else you can imagine. Have fun!

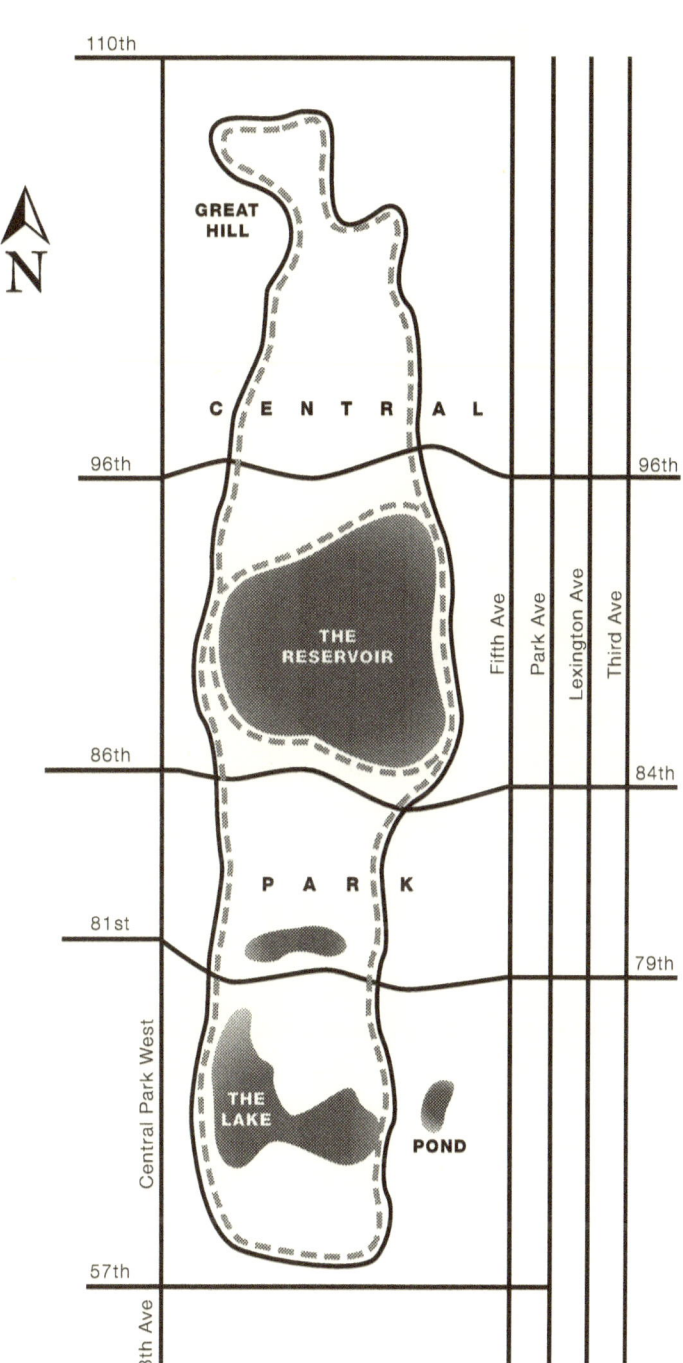

HUDSON RIVER

N

GREAT
HILL

C E N T R A L

110th

96th   96th

THE
RESERVOIR

Fifth Ave

Park Ave

Lexington Ave

Third Ave

86th   84th

P A R K

81st

79th

Central Park West

THE
LAKE

POND

57th

8th Ave

PORTLAND, OREGON

A green belt begins at the Burnside Bridge, just a couple of blocks from downtown Portland, and offers great running. Heading south, the bike path will take you through the Harbor Shopping Area. Run past the shopping area and continue south through an industrial and boat dry dock area. At the Spaghetti Factory Restaurant the bike trail will begin again and continues as far as you will want to run. The view of the Willamette River is spectacular. You won't want to miss this run.

Another interesting run is along Terwilliger Boulevard. You can park at Duniway Park to begin this run or run south through the Portland State Campus and, making a couple turns, you will arrive at Duniway Park. This park has a track you can warm up on, with a huge clock for timing your laps. About one block away is another interesting track that winds around and up and down to give you a quarter-mile lap. Fun! Anyway, the Terwilliger Boulevard Run starts here and continues mostly uphill for about three and a half miles. Don't worry, the forest is so beautiful along this route you'll hardly notice the climb.

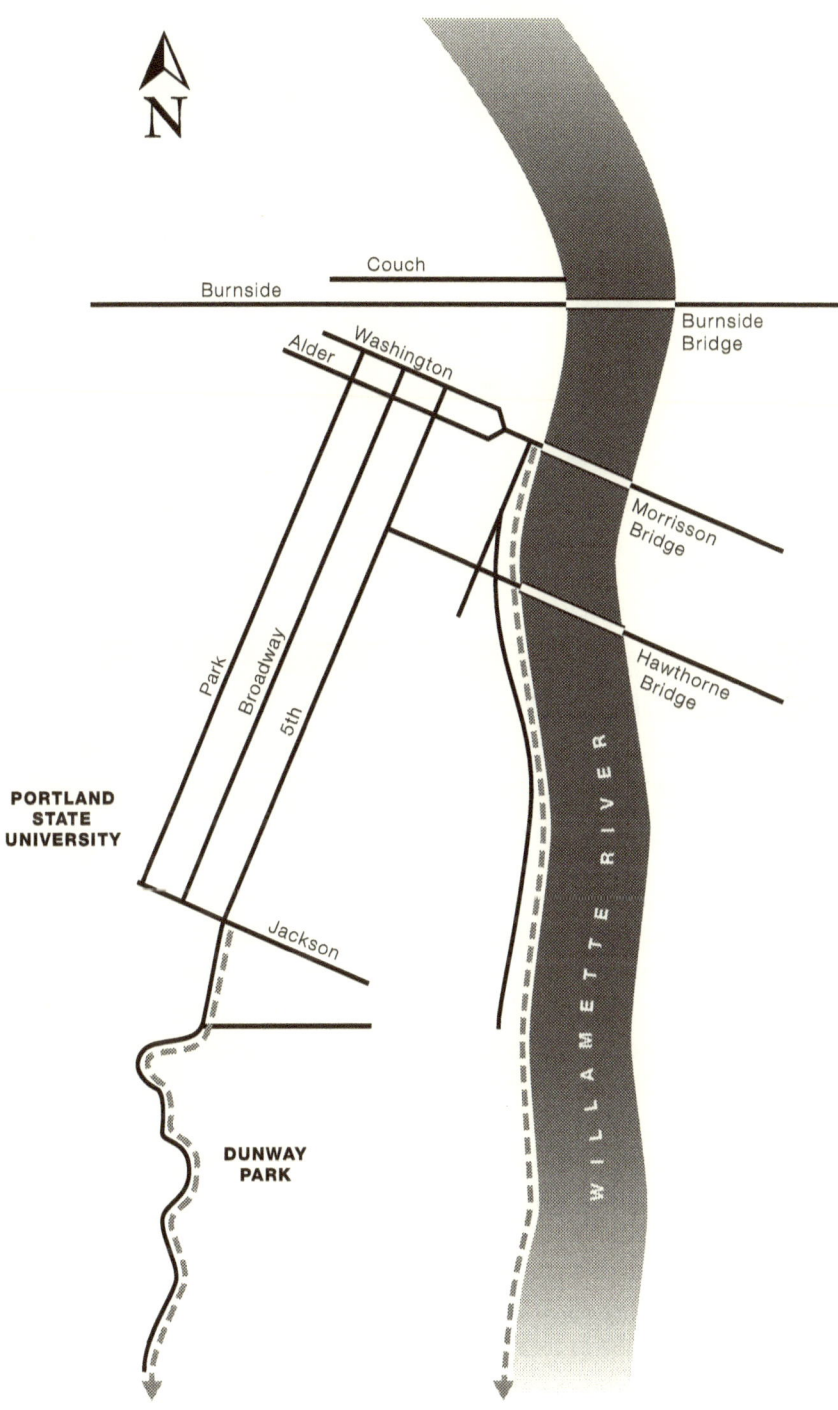

WASHINGTON, D.C.

In a city where the level of stress runs high, there is also a convenient and excellent place to reduce the pressure.

Between Constitution and Independence avenues you will find running paths that take you from the Capitol all the way to the Lincoln Memorial. A dirt footpath on both sides of the greenbelt will provide you with approximately a four-mile loop course. This is generally filled with runners during lunch break. Running along past the Washington and Lincoln memorials is so inspirational you'll probably want to take a side excursion on the way back and swing wide to include the Jefferson Memorial.

Two other runs you won't want to miss are in Rock Creek Park and along the Chesapeake and Ohio Canal. Both are easily accessible from Georgetown. Running in Rock Creek Park all the way up to the zoo, with several side excursions, you can easily run fifteen or more miles before you realize what you have done. Not to be outdone, the Chesapeake and Ohio Canal can lead you all the way, deep into Pennsylvania's countryside. Stick to the local area, just beyond the Francis Scott Key Bridge on the Potomac River, and you will be quite satisfied.

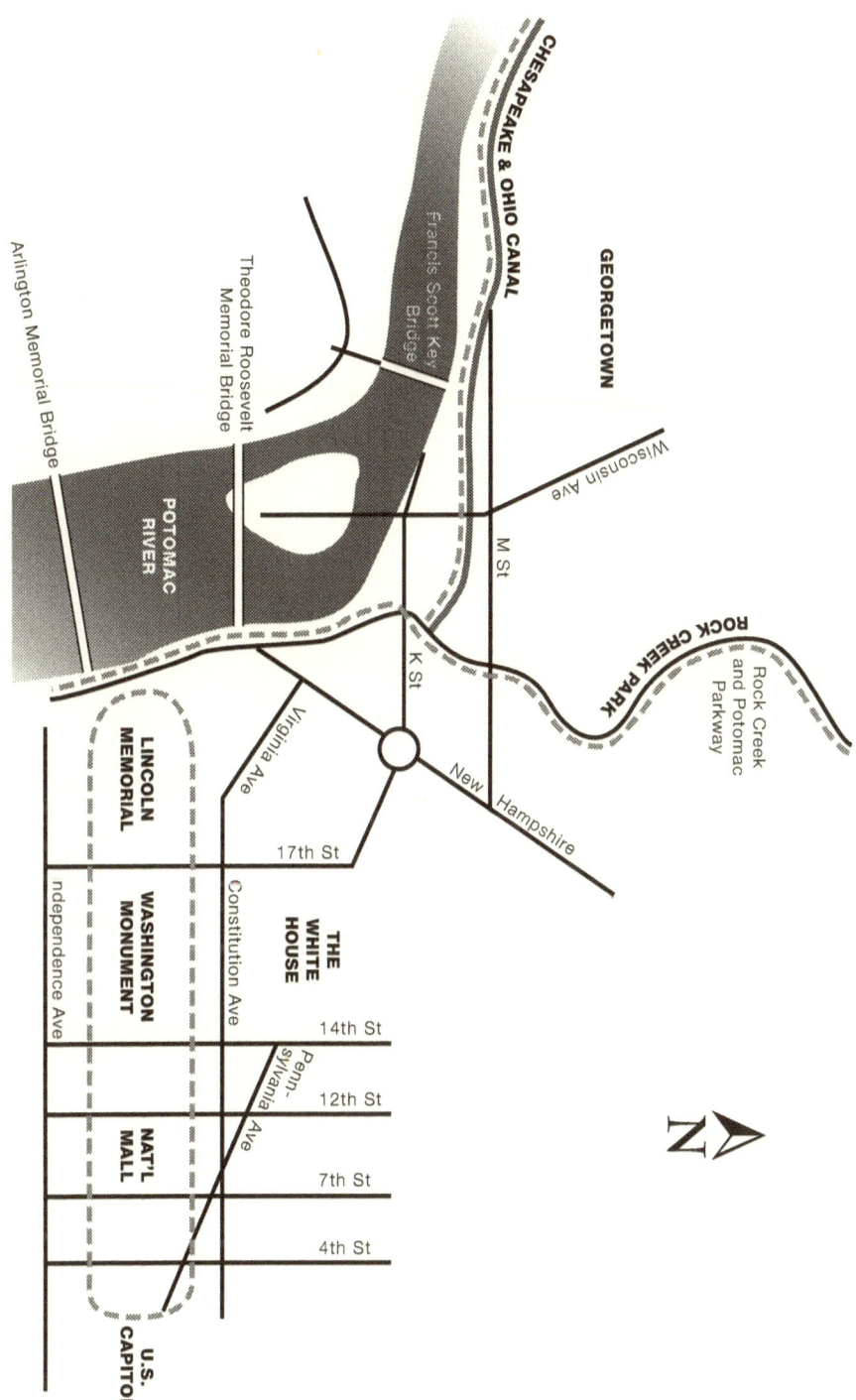

CHESAPEAKE & OHIO CANAL

GEORGETOWN

Francis Scott Key Bridge

Theodore Roosevelt Memorial Bridge

Arlington Memorial Bridge

Wisconsin Ave

M St

ROCK CREEK PARK

Rock Creek and Potomac Parkway

POTOMAC RIVER

K St

Virginia Ave

New Hampshire

LINCOLN MEMORIAL

17th St

Constitution Ave

Independence Ave

WASHINGTON MONUMENT

THE WHITE HOUSE

14th St

Penn-sylvania Ave

12th St

NAT'L MALL

7th St

4th St

U.S. CAPITOL

N

MILWAUKEE, WISCONSIN

If you like to run, this city will really offer you some spectacular mileage. Over seventy miles of trails surround this city—with scenery changing from the shores of Lake Michigan to the woods along the Menomonee River. I'll wager you could even find a beer when you're finished running!

With so many wonderful areas to run, you'll have to spend a week to enjoy all of them. Start with a run along the Milwaukee River that takes you through several parks on your trek. Next head south for a run, past Cudahy, on the Lake Michigan shoreline.

You are not done yet. Move west and spend a couple days running all the rivers and parks on the west side of town. Unbelievable running. Over twenty miles through the park system paralleling the Menomonee and Root rivers will keep you smiling.

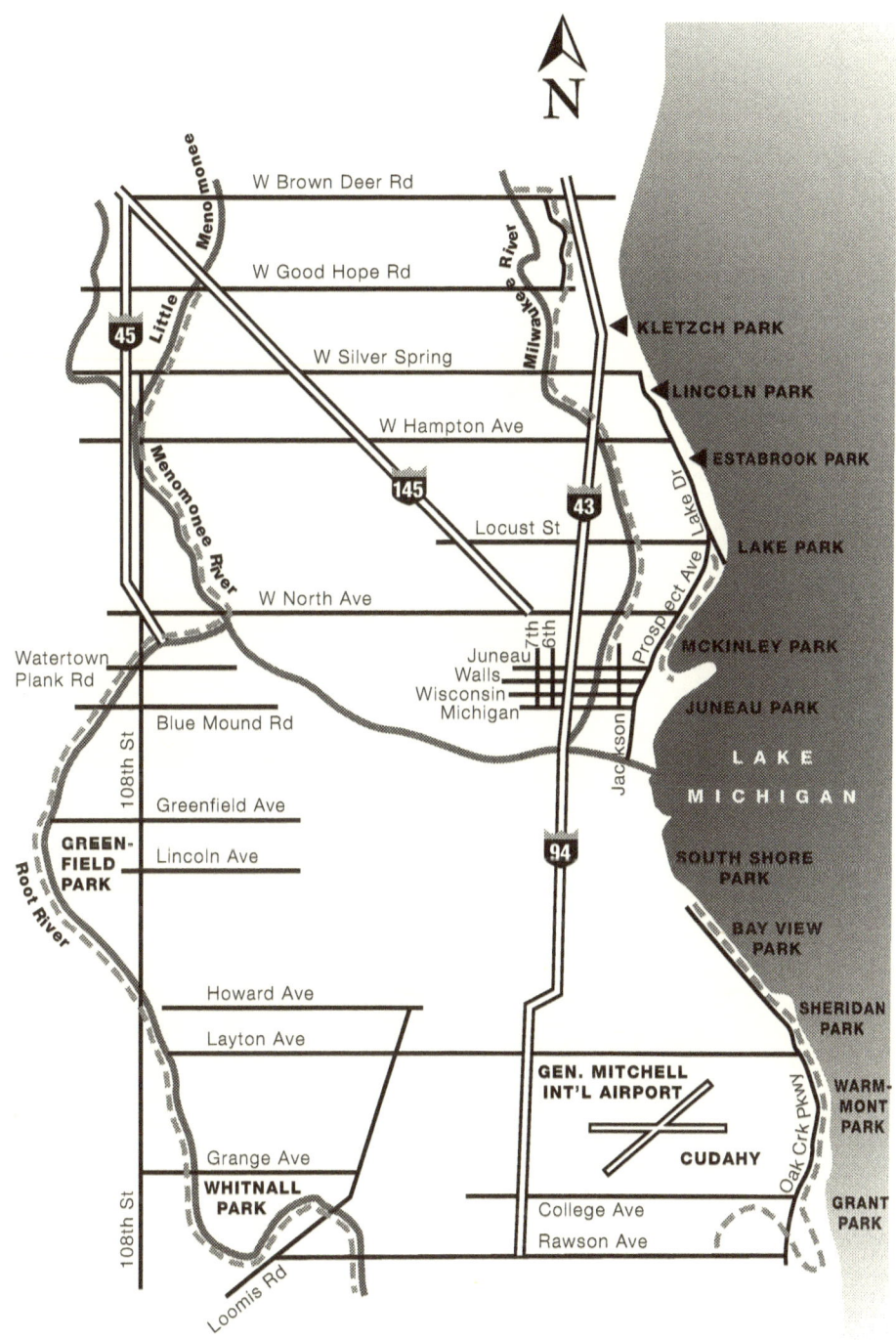

MINNEAPOLIS, MINNESOTA

I have seen great lake runs in many locales, but Minneapolis can offer you five beautiful lakes on one run. Perhaps this is why the Minneapolis Marathon, run in the fall, is always voted one of the greatest marathons. Five lakes to ponder, plus all the trees and birds—you'll be overwhelmed. If you have any energy left, you might attempt one more run along the mighty Mississippi. You won't regret it.

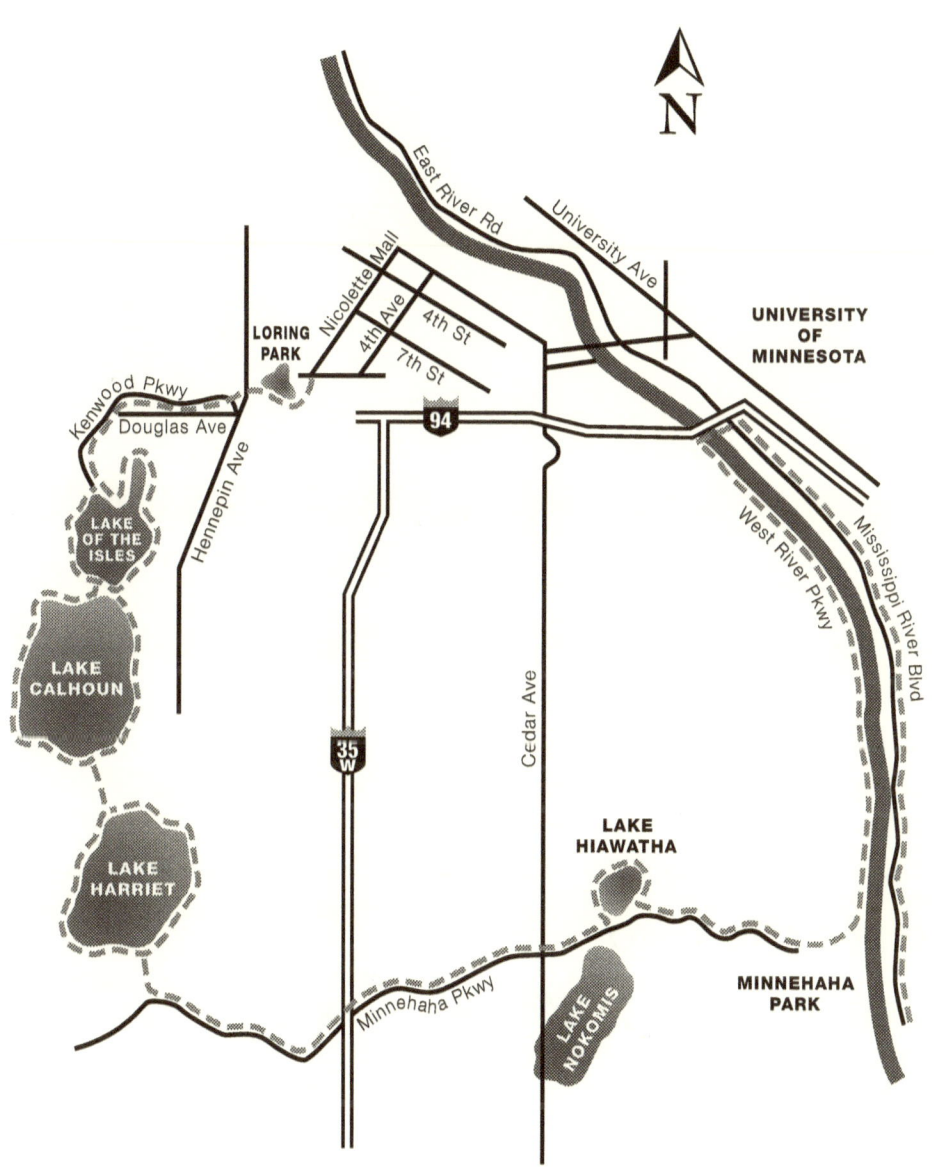

N

East River Rd

University Ave

Nicollette Mall

4th Ave

4th St

7th St

LORING
PARK

UNIVERSITY
OF
MINNESOTA

Kenwood Pkwy

Douglas Ave

Hennepin Ave

94

LAKE
OF THE
ISLES

West River Pkwy

Mississippi River Blvd

LAKE
CALHOUN

35
W

Cedar Ave

LAKE
HIAWATHA

LAKE
HARRIET

MINNEHAHA
PARK

Minnehaha Pkwy

LAKE
NOKOMIS

Great Runs

CLEVELAND, OHIO

Get your running shoes on and prepare yourself for the fantastic terrain of the Cleveland park system. The Rocky River Reservation boasts more than twenty miles of running trails along the Rocky River. It's a beautiful canyon setting, with trees and cliffs on both sides. Parks, golf courses, par courses, and picnic areas are plentiful.

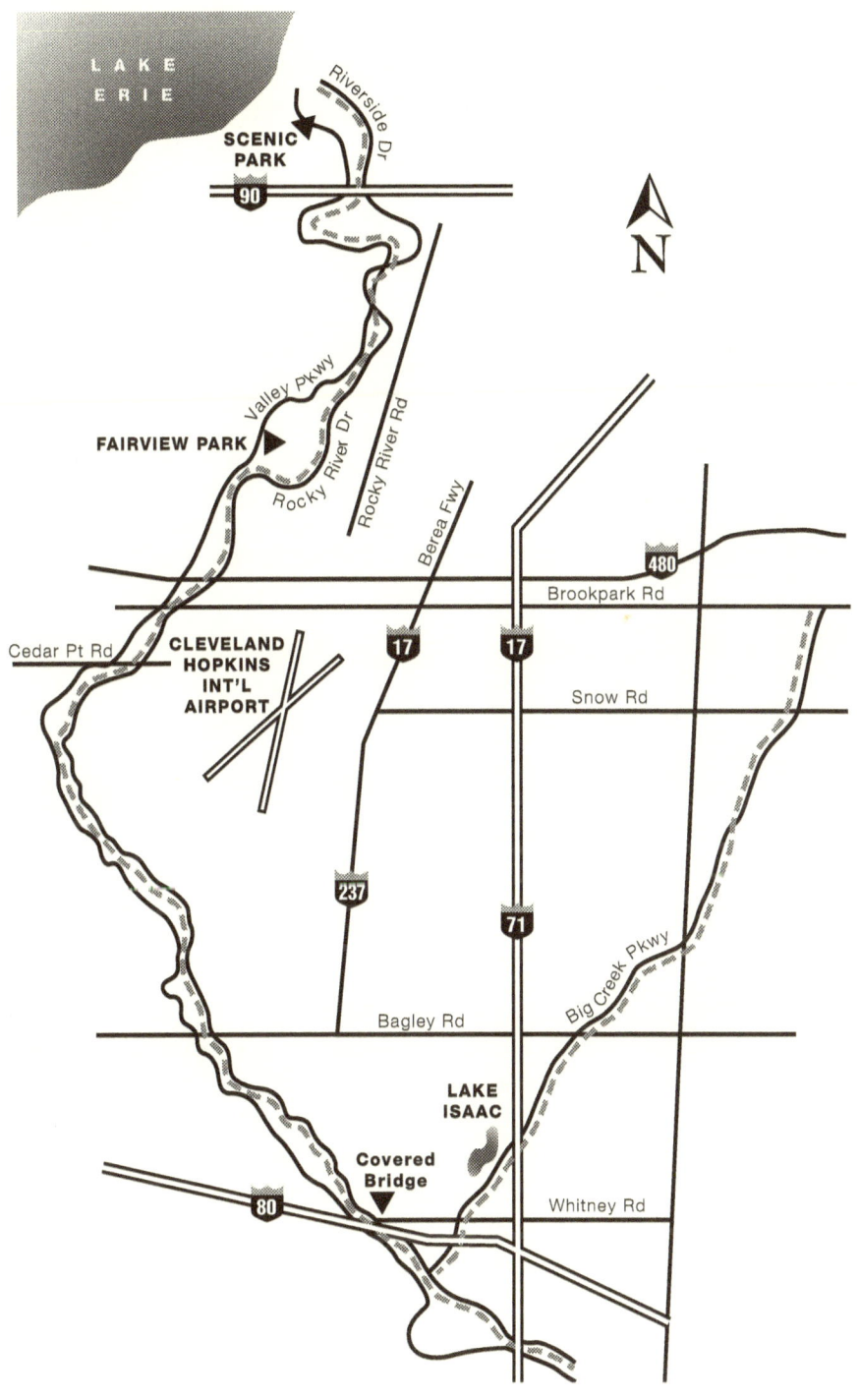

CHICAGO, ILLINOIS

In a city the size of Chicago, you would never imagine finding such convenient—not to mention excellent—places to run. The shoreline of Lake Michigan has many fabulous trails and parks. Starting at the south end of the park system, at Grand Avenue, you will experience a wonderful ten-mile (round trip) run past the city, boat harbors, beaches, gun clubs, and many parks. Turn around at Irving Park Road, just past the totem pole, and, on your return, take notice of everything you missed while you were northbound. Quite often you will experience a headwind running north, so take advantage of the wind at your back as you glance at all the magnificent buildings in the "windy city."

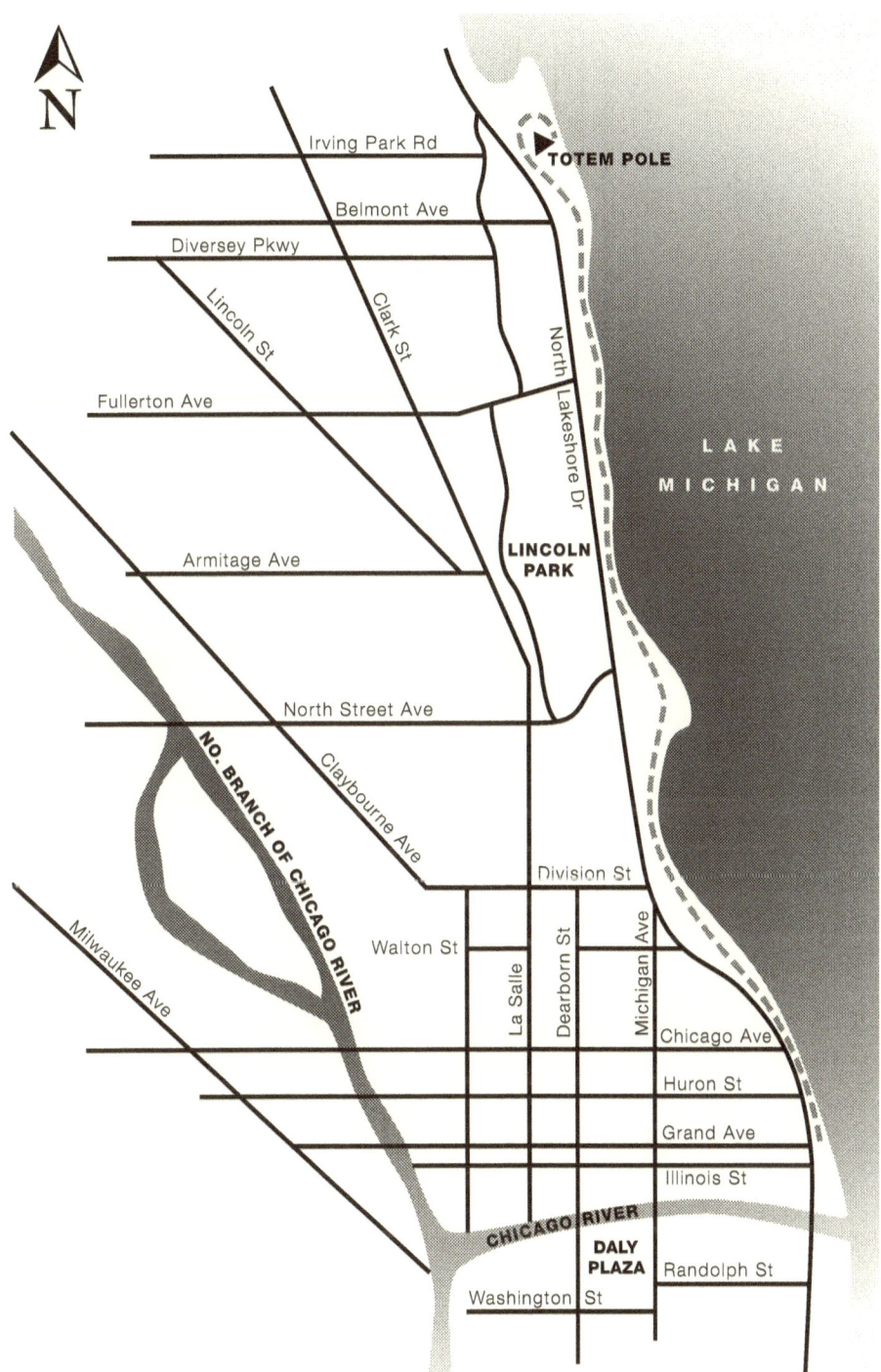

SAND POINT, IDAHO

Sandpoint prides itself on being a walking town, but running is also accepted. Many miles of bike trails thread through the city. A nice trail along Highway 2 will take you to Dover, about four miles. About one mile into this run you can turn right onto Syringa Road. This will take you about one mile through the woods before you'll want to turn right onto Ontario Street for another half a mile. Turn right again and you will come back to the bike trail. It's a nice change of pace and very peaceful.

Another interesting run will take you south to Sagle. Start at the Long Bridge. The first two miles will take you across Lake Pend Oreille. You can pick up the bike trail on the other side and continue for another two miles.

Before you leave town you have to run along the shoreline of Lake Pend Oreille. The start of this run is a little boring. Park at the old railway station and run north for about half a mile. Turn right and carefully cross the railroad tracks, looking for a secluded trail through the woods. This will take you to the shoreline trail and a great run of approximately four miles round trip.

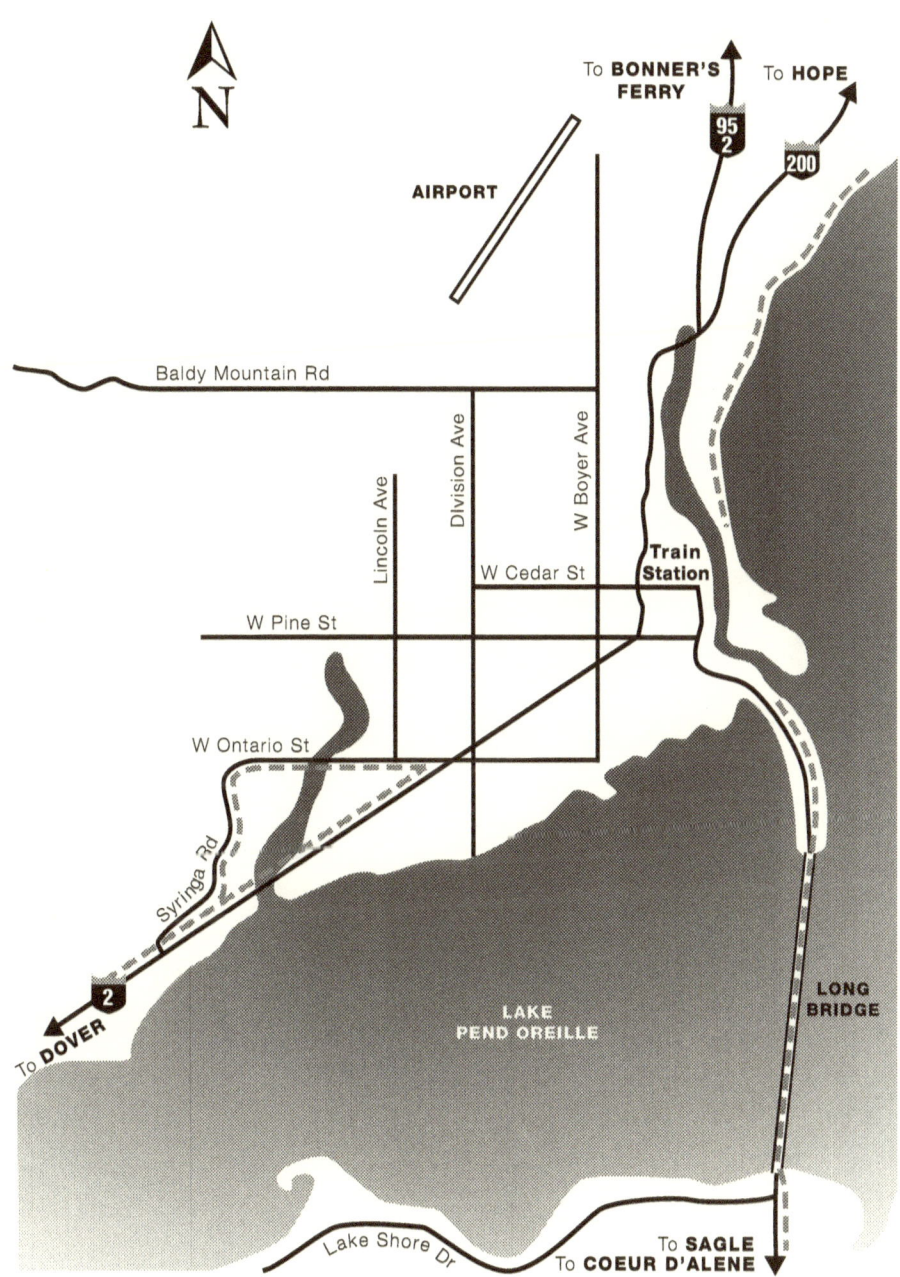

To **BONNER'S FERRY**

To **HOPE**

95
2

200

AIRPORT

Baldy Mountain Rd

Division Ave

W Boyer Ave

Lincoln Ave

Train Station

W Cedar St

W Pine St

W Ontario St

Syringa Rd

2

To **DOVER**

LAKE PEND OREILLE

LONG BRIDGE

Lake Shore Dr

To **SAGLE**
To **COEUR D'ALENE**

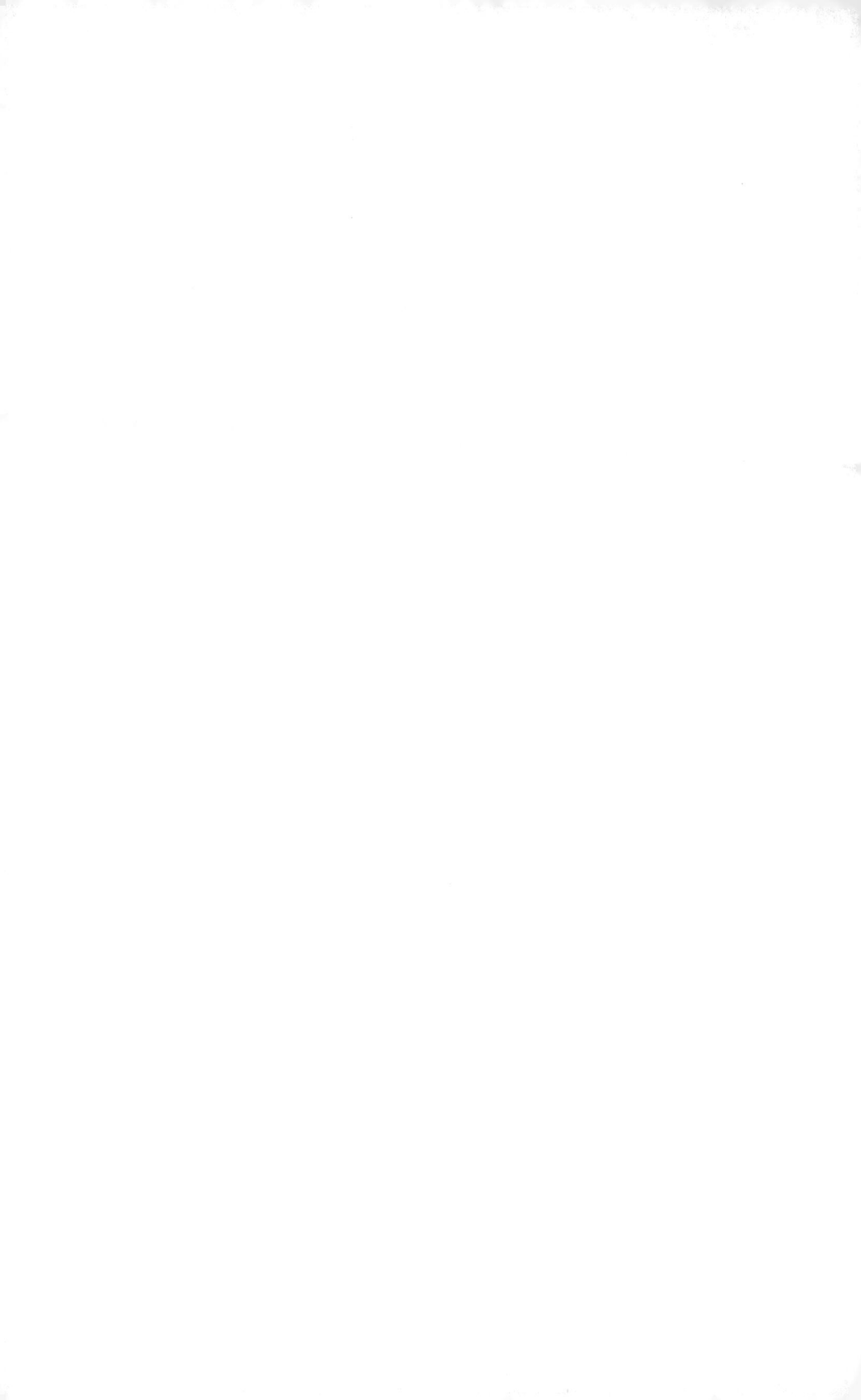

www.ingramcontent.com/pod-product-compliance
Lightning Source LLC
Chambersburg PA
CBHW031324290526
45784CB00014B/1142